Machine Learning/Deep Learning in Medical Image Processing

Machine Learning/Deep Learning in Medical Image Processing

Editor

Mizuho Nishio

MDPI • Basel • Beijing • Wuhan • Barcelona • Belgrade • Manchester • Tokyo • Cluj • Tianjin

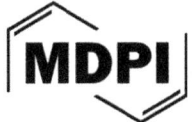

Editor
Mizuho Nishio
Kobe University and
Kyoto University
Japan

Editorial Office
MDPI
St. Alban-Anlage 66
4052 Basel, Switzerland

This is a reprint of articles from the Special Issue published online in the open access journal *Applied Sciences* (ISSN 2076-3417) (available at: https://www.mdpi.com/journal/applsci/special_issues/ML_Medical_Image).

For citation purposes, cite each article independently as indicated on the article page online and as indicated below:

LastName, A.A.; LastName, B.B.; LastName, C.C. Article Title. *Journal Name* **Year**, *Volume Number*, Page Range.

ISBN 978-3-0365-2664-5 (Hbk)
ISBN 978-3-0365-2665-2 (PDF)

© 2021 by the authors. Articles in this book are Open Access and distributed under the Creative Commons Attribution (CC BY) license, which allows users to download, copy and build upon published articles, as long as the author and publisher are properly credited, which ensures maximum dissemination and a wider impact of our publications.

The book as a whole is distributed by MDPI under the terms and conditions of the Creative Commons license CC BY-NC-ND.

Contents

About the Editor vii

Mizuho Nishio
Special Issue on "Machine Learning/Deep Learning in Medical Image Processing"
Reprinted from: *Appl. Sci.* **2021**, *11*, 11483, doi:10.3390/app112311483 1

Nikolaos Papandrianos and Elpiniki Papageorgiou
Automatic Diagnosis of Coronary Artery Disease in SPECT Myocardial Perfusion Imaging Employing Deep Learning
Reprinted from: *Appl. Sci.* **2021**, *11*, 6362, doi:10.3390/app11146362 3

Jinyoung Park, JaeJoon Hwang, Jihye Ryu, Inhye Nam, Sol-A Kim, Bong-Hae Cho, Sang-Hun Shin and Jae-Yeol Lee
Deep Learning Based Airway Segmentation Using Key Point Prediction
Reprinted from: *Appl. Sci.* **2021**, *11*, 3501, doi:10.3390/app11083501 27

Cristina L. Saratxaga, Jorge Bote, Juan F. Ortega-Morán, Artzai Picón, Elena Terradillos, Nagore Arbide del Río, Nagore Andraka, Estibaliz Garrote and Olga M. Conde
Characterization of Optical Coherence Tomography Images for Colon Lesion Differentiation under Deep Learning
Reprinted from: *Appl. Sci.* **2021**, *11*, 3119, doi:10.3390/app11073119 37

Francesco Martino, Domenico D. Bloisi, Andrea Pennisi, Mulham Fawakherji, Gennaro Ilardi, Daniela Russo, Daniele Nardi, Stefania Staibano, and Francesco Merolla
Deep Learning-Based Pixel-Wise Lesion Segmentation on Oral Squamous Cell Carcinoma Images
Reprinted from: *Appl. Sci.* **2020**, *10*, 8285, doi:10.3390/app10228285 57

Subrata Bhattacharjee, Cho-Hee Kim, Deekshitha Prakash, Hyeon-Gyun Park, Nam-Hoon Cho and Heung-Kook Choi
An Efficient Lightweight CNN and Ensemble Machine Learning Classification of Prostate Tissue Using Multilevel Feature Analysis
Reprinted from: *Appl. Sci.* **2020**, *10*, 8013, doi:10.3390/app10228013 71

Yasuyo Urase, Mizuho Nishio, Yoshiko Ueno, Atsushi K. Kono, Keitaro Sofue, Tomonori Kanda, Takaki Maeda, Munenobu Nogami, Masatoshi Hori and Takamichi Murakami
Simulation Study of Low-Dose Sparse-Sampling CT with Deep Learning-Based Reconstruction: Usefulness for Evaluation of Ovarian Cancer Metastasis
Reprinted from: *Appl. Sci.* **2020**, *10*, 4446, doi:10.3390/app10134446 95

Mizuho Nishio, Shunjiro Noguchi and Koji Fujimoto
Automatic Pancreas Segmentation Using Coarse-Scaled 2D Model of Deep Learning: Usefulness of Data Augmentation and Deep U-Net
Reprinted from: *Appl. Sci.* **2020**, *10*, 3360, doi:10.3390/app10103360 111

About the Editor

Mizuho Nishio currently serves as a program-specific assistant professor at the Department of Radiology in Kobe University Hospital, Kobe, Japan. In addition, he also works at the Department of Diagnostic Imaging and Nuclear Medicine in Kyoto University Hospital, Kyoto, Japan. His research area is the application of machine learning/deep learning to medical image analysis. Recently, he has focused on the automatic diagnosis of COVID-19 using deep learning on chest x-ray images. Dr. Nishio earned his medical degree from the Kobe University School of Medicine. He completed his radiology residency at Nishi-Kobe medical center in Kobe, where he received the Hospital's Award for installation of a picture archiving and communication system in the Department of Radiology. He obtained his Ph.D. degree from the Kobe University Graduate School of Medicine. After that, he served as program-specific assistant professors at the Department of Radiology in Kobe University Graduate School of Medicine and Kyoto University Hospital.

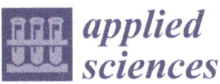

Editorial

Special Issue on "Machine Learning/Deep Learning in Medical Image Processing"

Mizuho Nishio

Department of Diagnostic Imaging and Nuclear Medicine, Kyoto University Graduate School of Medicine, 54 Kawahara-cho, Shogoin, Sakyo-ku, Kyoto 606-8507, Japan; nishiomizuho@gmail.com or nishio.mizuho.3e@kyoto-u.ac.jp; Tel.: +81-75-751-3760; Fax: +81-75-771-9709

Many recent studies on medical image processing have involved the use of machine learning (ML) and deep learning (DL) [1,2]. In ML, features are frequently extracted from medical images to aid in the interpretation of useful information. However, this process might hinder the images from being fully utilized. In contrast to ML, DL does not require such feature extractions. In fact, DL outperforms a combination of ML and feature extraction in computer vision [3]. Therefore, DL has been used more frequently in recent medical image studies.

This special issue, "Machine Learning/Deep Learning in Medical Image Processing", has been launched to provide an opportunity for researchers in the area of medical image processing to highlight recent developments made in their fields with ML/DL. Seven excellent papers that cover a wide variety of medical/clinical aspects are selected in this special issue [4–10]. Of these, four papers were related to radiology (computed tomography (CT) and nuclear medicine) and two were related to pathology (prostate carcinoma and oral squamous cell carcinoma). These seven papers have been summarized as follows:

- Nishio et al. proposed and evaluated a method for automatic pancreas segmentation from CT images [4]. Their method consists of a deep U-net and combinations of data augmentation, and is demonstrated to be superior to the baseline U-net and conventional data augmentation.
- Urase et al. proposed combining sparse-sampling CT with DL-based reconstruction to detect the metastases of malignant ovarian tumors [5]. Results demonstrate their method to be more useful in detecting metastases than the conventional residual encoder-decoder convolutional neural network (RED-CNN) method.
- Bhattacharjee et al. introduced two lightweight CNN architectures and an ensemble ML method for binary classification between the two grade groups of prostate tissue (benign vs. malignant) [6]. The classifications achieved by their models were promisingly accurate.
- Martino et al. investigated the tumor segmentation of pathology images [7]. Their important contribution was the construction of the Oral Cancer Annotated (ORCA) dataset [11], which contains ground-true data derived from the well-known Cancer Genome Atlas (TCGA) dataset [12].
- Saratxaga et al. proposed a DL model for the automatic classification (benign vs. malignant) of optical coherence tomography images obtained from colonic samples [8].
- Park et al. proposed a regression neural network-based DL model [9] to measure airway volume and investigated the accuracy of those measurements. Results showed a good correlation between the manual and model-based measurements.
- Papandrianos et al. proposed a DL model for the binary classification (normal vs. coronary artery disease) [10]. Single-photon-emission CT images of myocardial perfusions were the required inputs for this model and results demonstrate the efficacy of their DL model over existing models in nuclear medicine.

Citation: Nishio, M. Special Issue on "Machine Learning/Deep Learning in Medical Image Processing". *Appl. Sci.* **2021**, *11*, 11483. https://doi.org/10.3390/app112311483

Received: 5 November 2021
Accepted: 30 November 2021
Published: 3 December 2021

Publisher's Note: MDPI stays neutral with regard to jurisdictional claims in published maps and institutional affiliations.

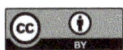

Copyright: © 2021 by the author. Licensee MDPI, Basel, Switzerland. This article is an open access article distributed under the terms and conditions of the Creative Commons Attribution (CC BY) license (https://creativecommons.org/licenses/by/4.0/).

These seven papers are expected to tremendously benefit readers in various aspects of medical image processing. I believe that this special issue contains a series of excellent research works on medical image processing with ML and DL.

Funding: JSPS KAKENHI (grant number: 19H03599 and JP19K17232).

Institutional Review Board Statement: Approval of institutional review board is not required.

Informed Consent Statement: Informed consent is not required.

Data Availability Statement: No data are used in this editorial.

Acknowledgments: I would like to thank the authors of the seven papers, the many reviewers, and the editorial team of *Applied Sciences*—especially the Assistant Managing Editor, Seraina Shi—for their valuable contributions towards making this special issue a success. For writing this editorial, the author was partly supported by JSPS KAKENHI (grant number: 19H03599 and JP19K17232).

Conflicts of Interest: The author declares no conflict of interest.

References

1. Yamashita, R.; Nishio, M.; Do, R.K.G.; Togashi, K. Convolutional neural networks: An overview and application in radiology. *Insights Imaging* **2018**, *9*, 611–629. [CrossRef] [PubMed]
2. Chartrand, G.; Cheng, P.M.; Vorontsov, E.; Drozdzal, M.; Turcotte, S.; Pal, C.J.; Kadoury, S.; Tang, A. Deep Learning: A Primer for Radiologists. *RadioGraphics* **2017**, *37*, 2113–2131. [CrossRef] [PubMed]
3. Russakovsky, O.; Deng, J.; Su, H.; Krause, J.; Satheesh, S.; Ma, S.; Huang, Z.; Karpathy, A.; Khosla, A.; Bernstein, M.; et al. ImageNet Large Scale Visual Recognition Challenge. *Int. J. Comput. Vis.* **2015**, *115*, 211–252. [CrossRef]
4. Nishio, M.; Noguchi, S.; Fujimoto, K. Automatic Pancreas Segmentation Using Coarse-Scaled 2D Model of Deep Learning: Usefulness of Data Augmentation and Deep U-Net. *Appl. Sci.* **2020**, *10*, 3360. [CrossRef]
5. Urase, Y.; Nishio, M.; Ueno, Y.; Kono, A.; Sofue, K.; Kanda, T.; Maeda, T.; Nogami, M.; Hori, M.; Murakami, T. Simulation Study of Low-Dose Sparse-Sampling CT with Deep Learning-Based Reconstruction: Usefulness for Evaluation of Ovarian Cancer Metastasis. *Appl. Sci.* **2020**, *10*, 4446. [CrossRef]
6. Bhattacharjee, S.; Kim, C.H.; Prakash, D.; Park, H.G.; Cho, N.H.; Choi, H.K. An Efficient Lightweight CNN and Ensemble Machine Learning Classification of Prostate Tissue Using Multilevel Feature Analysis. *Appl. Sci.* **2020**, *10*, 8013. [CrossRef]
7. Martino, F.; Bloisi, D.D.; Pennisi, A.; Fawakherji, M.; Ilardi, G.; Russo, D.; Nardi, D.; Staibano, S.; Merolla, F. Deep Learning-Based Pixel-Wise Lesion Segmentation on Oral Squamous Cell Carcinoma Images. *Appl. Sci.* **2020**, *10*, 8285. [CrossRef]
8. Saratxaga, C.; Bote, J.; Ortega-Morán, J.; Picón, A.; Terradillos, E.; del Río, N.; Andraka, N.; Garrote, E.; Conde, O. Characterization of Optical Coherence Tomography Images for Colon Lesion Differentiation under Deep Learning. *Appl. Sci.* **2021**, *11*, 3119. [CrossRef]
9. Park, J.; Hwang, J.; Ryu, J.; Nam, I.; Kim, S.-A.; Cho, B.-H.; Shin, S.-H.; Lee, J.-Y. Deep Learning Based Airway Segmentation Using Key Point Prediction. *Appl. Sci.* **2021**, *11*, 3501. [CrossRef]
10. Papandrianos, N.; Papageorgiou, E. Automatic Diagnosis of Coronary Artery Disease in SPECT Myocardial Perfusion Imaging Employing Deep Learning. *Appl. Sci.* **2021**, *11*, 6362. [CrossRef]
11. ORCA Dataset. Available online: https://sites.google.com/unibas.it/orca (accessed on 3 December 2021).
12. The Cancer Genome Atlas Program—National Cancer Institute. Available online: https://www.cancer.gov/about-nci/organization/ccg/research/structural-genomics/tcga (accessed on 3 December 2021).

Article

Automatic Diagnosis of Coronary Artery Disease in SPECT Myocardial Perfusion Imaging Employing Deep Learning

Nikolaos Papandrianos * and Elpiniki Papageorgiou

Department of Energy Systems, Faculty of Technology, University of Thessaly, Geopolis Campus, Larissa-Trikala Ring Road, 41500 Larissa, Greece; elpinikipapageorgiou@uth.gr
* Correspondence: npapandrianos@uth.gr

Abstract: Focusing on coronary artery disease (CAD) patients, this research paper addresses the problem of automatic diagnosis of ischemia or infarction using single-photon emission computed tomography (SPECT) (Siemens Symbia S Series) myocardial perfusion imaging (MPI) scans and investigates the capabilities of deep learning and convolutional neural networks. Considering the wide applicability of deep learning in medical image classification, a robust CNN model whose architecture was previously determined in nuclear image analysis is introduced to recognize myocardial perfusion images by extracting the insightful features of an image and use them to classify it correctly. In addition, a deep learning classification approach using transfer learning is implemented to classify cardiovascular images as normal or abnormal (ischemia or infarction) from SPECT MPI scans. The present work is differentiated from other studies in nuclear cardiology as it utilizes SPECT MPI images. To address the two-class classification problem of CAD diagnosis, achieving adequate accuracy, simple, fast and efficient CNN architectures were built based on a CNN exploration process. They were then employed to identify the category of CAD diagnosis, presenting its generalization capabilities. The results revealed that the applied methods are sufficiently accurate and able to differentiate the infarction or ischemia from healthy patients (overall classification accuracy = 93.47% ± 2.81%, AUC score = 0.936). To strengthen the findings of this study, the proposed deep learning approaches were compared with other popular state-of-the-art CNN architectures for the specific dataset. The prediction results show the efficacy of new deep learning architecture applied for CAD diagnosis using SPECT MPI scans over the existing ones in nuclear medicine.

Keywords: coronary artery disease; SPECT MPI scans; deep learning; convolutional neural networks; transfer learning; classification models

Citation: Papandrianos, N.; Papageorgiou, E. Automatic Diagnosis of Coronary Artery Disease in SPECT Myocardial Perfusion Imaging Employing Deep Learning. *Appl. Sci.* **2021**, *11*, 6362. https://doi.org/10.3390/app11146362

Academic Editor: Mizuho Nishio

Received: 20 May 2021
Accepted: 7 July 2021
Published: 9 July 2021

Publisher's Note: MDPI stays neutral with regard to jurisdictional claims in published maps and institutional affiliations.

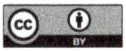

Copyright: © 2021 by the authors. Licensee MDPI, Basel, Switzerland. This article is an open access article distributed under the terms and conditions of the Creative Commons Attribution (CC BY) license (https://creativecommons.org/licenses/by/4.0/).

1. Introduction

Coronary artery disease (CAD) is one of the most frequent pathological conditions and the primary cause of death worldwide [1]. Described by its inflammatory nature [2], CAD is an atherosclerotic disease usually developed by the interaction of genetic and environmental factors [3] and leads to cardiovascular events including stable angina, unstable angina, myocardial infarction (MI), or sudden cardiac death [4]. Coronary heart disease (CHD) has a significant impact on mortality and morbidity in Europe, whereas its management requires a large proportion of national healthcare budgets. Thus, an accurate CAD (ischemia, infarction, etc.) diagnosis is crucial on a socioeconomic level. CAD diagnosis usually requires the implementation of suitable diagnostic imaging [5,6]. In this direction, non-invasive imaging techniques are the most preferred methods for diagnosing CAD, prognostication, selection for revascularization and assessing acute coronary syndromes [7]. Even though they have raised the direct expenditure regarding investigation, they are likely to reduce overall costs, leading to greater cost-effectiveness [7].

To achieve a reliable and cost-effective CAD diagnosis, a variety of modern imaging techniques such as single-photon emission computed tomography (SPECT) myocardial perfusion imaging (MPI), positron emission tomography (PET), and cardiovascular computed tomography (CT) have been utilized in clinical practice [8–12]. According to the EANM guidelines [13], radionuclide MPI with the contribution of SPECT imaging is a remarkably efficient technique regarding the CAD diagnosis [14,15].

Myocardial perfusion scintigraphy (MPS) is a well-established, non-invasive imaging technique proven effective in diagnosing angina and myocardial infarction. Specifically, SPECT MPI depicts the information regarding the spreading of a radioactive compound within the heart in three dimensions and is considered the most frequently performed procedure in nuclear cardiology [16]. Among others, it is used for predicting future CAD events and identifying coronary artery disease severity. Regarding the detection of myocardial ischemia, MPS outperforms ECG in terms of accuracy [7,17]. Furthermore, applying the MPS imaging method reduces the number of angiographies, offering proper treatment planning [18].

In the discipline of cardiovascular imaging using nuclear cardiology techniques, Slart et al. explored the notion regarding the deployment of artificial intelligence (AI) based on modern machine learning, focusing on methods and computational models currently used [19]. The goal is to enhance diagnostic performance through complex image analysis and interpretation [20]. However, image interpretation is a demanding yet time-consuming task which relies mainly on physicians' experience [21]. On this basis, interpretation can be standardized with the contribution of CAD tools providing enhanced overall objectivity. The diagnostic accuracy is also improved, whereas the diagnostic time and healthcare costs are significantly reduced. Since there is an extensive existing and standardized imaging database in the realm of nuclear cardiac imaging, AI becomes the right candidate to be utilized in this domain [22]. More specifically, AI is currently spreading throughout three main areas related to cardiac SPECT/CT and PET/CT imaging. These involve the processes of automation of image detection and segmentation, spotting patients suffering from obstructive coronary artery disease (CAD), and risk assessment of coronary syndromes [23]. Overall, computer-aided diagnosis can serve as a supportive tool that can assist not only in the realization of unusual and difficult medical cases but to train inexperienced clinical staff too [23].

Computer-aided diagnosis is well attained through the deployment of machine learning, including deep learning algorithms, which are characterized by an extraordinary capability for medical image interpretation in the realm of medical image analysis [24–27]. Acknowledging that deep learning has shown remarkable efficacy in visual object detection and classification, researchers are highly intrigued by the capabilities that deep learning tools possess for improving the accuracy of CAD classification, helping nuclear physicians in this direction [28–30].

1.1. Deep Learning in Image Analysis

In the domain of medical imaging, deep learning is mainly implemented by convolutional neural networks (CNNs) [25,31–33], which are considered an efficient and dynamic approach for extracting features concerning image classification and segmentation tasks. Before CNN development, this process had to be accomplished using insufficient machine learning models or by hand. However, after their entrance into medical imaging, CNNs could use these features that had been learned directly from the data. Among the marked characteristics of CNNs is their capability of analyzing and classifying images, making them powerful deep learning models for image analysis [24,25,32,34]. CNN resembles a standard artificial neural network (ANN) in its characteristics, utilizing backpropagation and gradient descent for training. However, more pooling layers and layers of convolutions are present concerning its structure.

Among the most common CNNs methods in medical image analysis, there are:

AlexNet (2012): Developed by Yann LeCun et al. [35], this network has a similar architecture to LeNet [36] but consists of more filters per layer, including stacked convolutional layers. Its specifications include $11 \times 11, 5 \times 5, 3 \times 3$ convolutions, max pooling, dropout, data augmentation, rectified linear unit (ReLU) activations and stochastic gradient descent (SGD) with momentum [37]. It attaches ReLU activations after each layer, either convolutional or fully connected. The deep learning boom was attributed to AlexNet, when this architecture won the 2012 ILSVRC competition by a considerable margin. Some features worth mentioning are the computational split among many GPUs, dropout regularization, data augmentation, and the ReLU activation function.

ZFNet (2013): This network constitutes a minor adaptation of AlexNet and won the 2013 ILSVRC competition [38].

VGGNet16 (2014): This network incorporates 16 convolutional layers and is popular due to its consistent structure [39]. Being similar to AlexNet, this model presents only 3×3 convolutions but comprises many filters. Currently, VGGNet16 is the most preferred choice in the community for feature extraction from images. At the same time, it gave great popularity to the notion of creating deeper networks by using smaller filter kernels [40].

GoogleNet: It involves a standard piled convolutional layer and one or more fully connected layers [41]. Inception modules were also introduced, applying different-sized filters to the input and concatenated in the end. This way, the module can extract different levels of features simultaneously. Another notion introduced by GoogleNet, which won the 2014 ILSVRC competition, was that there is a global average pooling instead of fully connected layers in the network's ending, reducing the model parameters.

ResNet (2015): This type of CNN architecture introduced the "identity shortcut connection" to handle the well-known "vanishing gradients" issue that characterizes deep networks. This technique revealed that extremely deep networks could use standard SGD along with residual modules for their training [42].

DenseNet (2017): Being another important CNN architecture, DenseNet outweighs other networks as it sorted out the gradient vanishment problem by directly connecting all its layers. Meanwhile, feature delivery is optimized; therefore, it can make more efficient use of it. It is a widespread technique for disease diagnosis, and more recently, it efficiently addressed the task of cardiac disease classification, as reported in [43].

1.2. Machine Learning and Deep Learning in SPECT Nuclear Cardiology Imaging

Currently, regarding SPECT MPI, which is one of the established methods for imaging in nuclear cardiology, researchers face the challenge of developing an algorithm that can automatically characterize the status of the patients with known or suspected coronary artery disease. The accuracy of this algorithm needs to be extreme due to the importance of people's lives. Since deep learning algorithms have the capacity to improve the accuracy of CAD screening, they have been broadly explored in the domain of nuclear cardiovascular imaging analysis.

ML and DL methods have both been explored to assess the likelihood of obstructive CAD. In the context of ML algorithms for CAD diagnosis, ANN, SVM and boosted ensemble methods have been investigated. In a single-center study for the detection of obstructive CAD, ML was utilized with SPECT myocardial perfusion imaging (MPI) combining clinical data of 1181 patients and provided AUC values (0.94 ± 0.01), which were significantly better than total perfusion deficit (0.88 ± 0.01) or visual readout [44].

ML was also explored in the multi-center REFINE SPECT (REgistry of Fast Myocardial Perfusion Imaging with NExt generation SPECT) registry [45]. In this study, 1980 patients of possible CAD went through a stress/rest 99mTc-sestamibi/tetrofosmin MPI. The ML algorithm embedding 18 clinical, 9 stress test, and 28 imaging variables from 1980 patients produced an AUC of 0.79 [0.77, 0.80], which is higher than that regarding (TPD) 0.71 [0.70, 0.73] or ischemic TPD 0.72 [0.71, 0.74] in the prediction of early coronary revascularization.

In [46], ANN was applied for interpreting MPS with suspected myocardial ischemia and infarction on 418 patients who underwent ECG-gated MPS at a single hospital. The ANN-based method was compared against a conventional automated quantification software package. The results showed that the model based on neural networks presents interpretations more similar to experienced clinicians than the other method examined.

Using clinical and other quantification data, the authors of [47] deployed the boosted ensemble machine learning algorithm and the ANN, achieving classification accuracy of up to 90%. SVMs have been exploited in [48] and have been trained considering a group of 957 patients with either correlating invasive coronary angiography or a low possibility of CAD. The AUC value produced for SVM classifier combining quantitative perfusion (TPD and ISCH) and functional data was as high as 86%.

Moreover, several recent research studies explore ML and DL methods for diagnosing CAD in nuclear cardiology using polar maps instead of SPECT MPI scans. The studies devoted to polar maps are set out as follows: in [49], Perfex and an ANN are used with polar maps, while in [50–52], polar maps were utilized along with DL methods. In [49], polar maps of stress and rest examinations of 243 patients who underwent SPECT and coronary angiography within three months were used as input images to train ANN models. The produced AUC results of receiver operating characteristics (ROC) analysis for neural networks was 0.74, surpassing the corresponding AUC for other physicians.

Regarding the application of DL for CAD prediction, the authors in [50] employed deep learning, which was trained using polar maps, for predicting obstructive disease from myocardial perfusion imaging (MPI). The outcome is an improved automatic interpretation of MPI comparing to the total perfusion deficit (TPD). As a result, a pseudo-probability of CAD was deployed per vessel region and per individual patient. An AUC value of 0.80 was calculated concerning the detection of 70% stenosis or higher, still outperforming TPD. The DL procedure automatically predicted CAD from 2-view (upright and supine) polar maps data obtained from dedicated cardiac scanners in 1160 patients, improving current perfusion analysis in the prediction of obstructive CAD [50].

The same team of authors presented another interesting application of DL in the prediction of CAD. A three-fold feature extraction convolutional layer joined with three fully connected layers was deployed to analyze SPECT myocardial perfusion clinical data and polar maps from 1638 patients [51]. These scientific works have investigated the integration of clinical and imaging data and show how to formulate new autonomous systems for the automatic interpretation of SPECT and PET images. The authors in [52] proposed a graph-based convolutional neural network (GCNN) which used Chebyshev polynomials, achieving the highest accuracy (91%) compared with other neural-network-based methods.

Recently, authors in [53] were the first to study CAD diagnosis using solely SPECT MPI scans in deep learning. They developed two different classification models. The first one is based on deep learning (DL), while the second is based on knowledge to classify MPI scans into two types automatically, ischemia or healthy, exclusively employing the SPECT MPI scans at the input level. Performing exploitation of the well-known DL methods in medical image analysis (such as AlexNet, GoogleNet, ResNet, DenseNet, VGG16, VGG19), the best DL model was determined to be VGG16 with support vector machine (SVM) deep features shallow, concerning classification accuracy. The first model to be developed exploits different pre-trained deep neural networks (DNNs) along with the traditional classifier SVM with the deep and shallow features extracted from various pre-trained DNNs for the classification task. The knowledge-based model, in its turn, is focused on converting the knowledge extracted from experts in the domain into proper image processing methods such as color thresholding, segmentation, feature extraction and some heuristics to classify SPECT images. First, the images were divided into six segments (A, B, C, D, E, F), and the features were extracted from each segment to measure the shapes. Next, a classification rule set assigned by experts was applied. The parameters were empirically identified and fine-tuned on the training and validation images. The produced overall 2-class classification accuracy was 93% for both methods.

As has emerged from the related literature regarding SPECT MPI, PET and PET-CT [54], a system based on deep learning provides similar performance to a nuclear physician in standalone mode. However, the overall performance is notably improved when it is used as a supportive tool for the physician [33,55–58]. Although SPECT MPI scans are of high importance for diagnosing CAD in nuclear cardiology, only one study was reported in the literature to apply CNNs in these types of MPI images. Thus, there is plenty of space for further research over the investigation on the advantageous and outstanding capabilities of CNNs in the field of nuclear cardiology.

1.3. Contribution of This Research Work

According to the previous work of the authors, new, fast and powerful CNN architectures were proposed to classify bone scintigraphy images for prostate and breast cancer patients in nuclear medicine [33,56,57,59]. More specifically, an RGB-based CNN model has been proposed to automatically identify whether a patient has bone metastasis or not by viewing whole-body scans. The results showed the superior performance of the RGB-CNN model against other state-of-the-art CNN models in this field [56,57]. Based on the advantageous features of the model, such as robustness, efficacy, low time cost, simple architecture, and training with a relatively small dataset [57], along with the promising results, authors were driven to study further and test the generalization capabilities of this methodology. This research work investigates the performance of the new models, applying them in nuclear cardiology, making the necessary parameterization and regularization to address the recognition of myocardial perfusion imaging from SPECT scans of patients with ischemia or infarction. Hence, the objectives are: (i) to diagnose cardiovascular disease by exploring efficient and robust CNN-based methods and (ii) to evaluate their performance, in line with SPECT MPI scans. A straightforward comparative analysis between the proposed RGB-based CNN methods with state-of-the-art deep learning methods, such as VGG16, Densenet, Mobilenet, etc., found in the literature was also conducted to show their classification performance. The produced results reveal that the proposed deep learning models achieve high classification accuracy with small datasets in SPECT MPI analysis and could show the path to future research directions with a view to a further investigation of the classification method application to other malignant medical states.

Overall, the innovation of this paper which highlights its contribution is two-fold: (a) the application of a predefined CNN-based structure, namely RGB-CNN [56,57], which was recently proposed in bone scintigraphy after a meticulous exploration analysis on its architecture and (b) the implementation of a deep learning classification model utilizing transfer learning for improving CAD diagnosis. The produced fast, robust and highly efficient model, in terms of accuracy and AUC score, can be applied to automatically identify patients with known or suspected coronary artery disease by looking at SPECT MPI scans.

This work is structured as follows: Section 2 includes the methods and materials used in this study. Section 3 provides the proposed deep learning architectures for SPECT MPI classification. In Section 4, a rigorous analysis is conducted, including the exploration of different configurations to determine the most accurate of the proposed classification models. Finally, the discussion of results and the conclusions follow in Section 5.

2. Materials and Methods

2.1. Patients and Imaging Protocol

The dataset used in this study corresponds to a retrospective review that includes 224 patients (age 32–85, average age 64.5, 65% men and 55% CAD), whose SPECT MPI scans were issued by the Nuclear Medicine Department of the Diagnostic Medical Center "Diagnostiko-Iatriki A.E.", Larisa, Greece. The dataset consists of images from patients who had undergone stress and rest SPECT MPI on suspicion of ischemia or infarction concerning the prediction of CAD between June 2013 and June 2017. The participant patients went through invasive coronary angiography (ICA) 40 days after MPI.

The set of stress and rest images collected from the records of 224 patients constitute the dataset used in this retrospective study. The dataset includes eight patients with infarction, 142 patients with ischemia, and eight patients with both infarction and ischemia, while the remaining (61 patients) were normal. Indicative image samples are illustrated in

Figure 1. This dataset is available only under request to the nuclear medicine physician and only for research purposes.

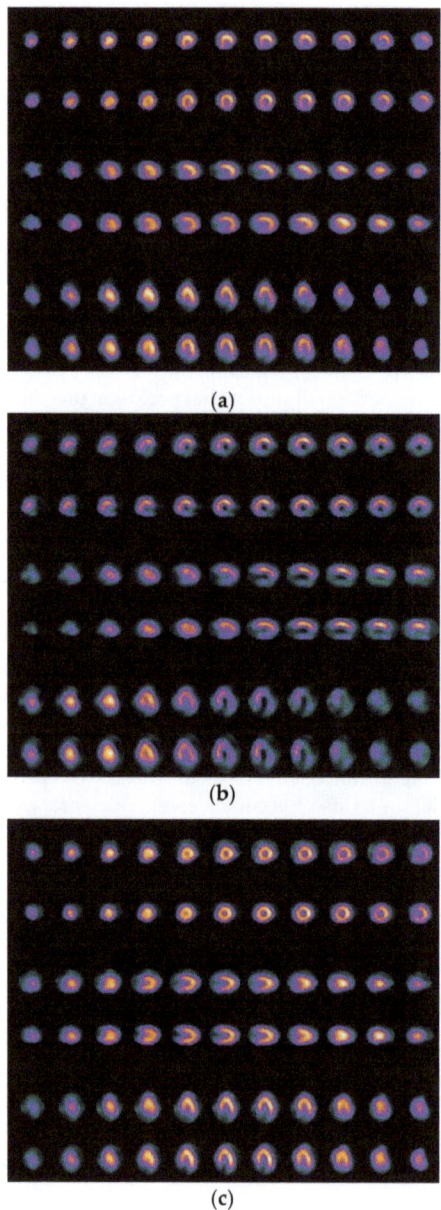

Figure 1. Image samples of SPECT MPI (from our dataset) (Labels: (a) ischemia, (b) infarction, (c) healthy).

A 1-day stress–rest injection protocol was used for Tc-99m tetrofosmin SPECT imaging. Patients underwent either symptom-limited Bruce protocol treadmill exercise testing (n = 154 [69%]) or pharmacologic stress (n = 69 [31%]) with radiotracer injection at peak exercise or during maximal hyperemia, respectively.

Within 20 min after an injection of 7 to 9 mCi 99mTc-tetrofosmin, stress SPECT images were collected due to either an effort test or pharmacological stress with dipyridamole. In the case of the effort test, a treadmill test was performed. The Bruce protocol was employed, and when at least 85% of the age-predicted maximum heart rate was achieved, a 99mTc-tetrofosmin injection was provided to the patient, whereas the exercise stopped 1 min later. Rest imaging followed 40 min after a dose of 21–27 mCi 99mTc-tetrofosmin had been injected. The data collected from SPECT system came from 32 projections regarding a period of 30 s for the stress and 30 s for the rest SPECT MPI. The rest of the configurations regarded a 140 keV photopeak, a 180-degree arc and a 64 × 64 matrix.

2.2. Visual Assessment

The assignment of patients' scanning was delivered by a Siemens gamma camera Symbia S series SPECT System (by dedicated workstation and software Syngo VE32B, Siemens Healthcare GmbH, Enlargen, Germany) comprising two heads that include low energy high-resolution (LEHR) collimators. The Syngo software was utilized for the Standard SPECT MPI processing allowing the nuclear medicine specialist to automatically produce SA (short axis), HLA (long horizontal axis), and VLA (long vertical axis) slices from raw data [55]. Afterwards, two expert readers with considerable clinical expertise in nuclear cardiology (N. Papandrianos, who is the first author of this work and N. Papathanasiou, who is Ass. Professor in Nuclear Medicine, University Hospital of Patras), provided visual assessments solely for the series of stress and rest perfusion images in color scale, though not including functional and clinical data [18]. The case is labeled as normal when there is a homogeneous involvement of 99mTc-tetrofosmin in the left ventricular walls.

On the contrary, a defect is defined when radiopharmaceuticals are less involved in any part of the myocardium. A comparative visual analysis is conducted, including the images collected after the stress SPECT MPI and those after the rest SPECT MPI, respectively. Potential defects are identified as a result of the injected radiopharmaceutical agent or even exercise. In this context, the condition is described as ischemia when a perfusion defect was detected in the SPECT images obtained after exercise but not in the rest images. Instead, infarction is the condition in which both stress and rest images include evidence of the defect. The classification process of all SPECT MPI images carried out by expert readers utilizes a two-class label (1 denotes normal and 2 abnormal) to administer additional tasks [53].

2.3. Overview of Convolutional Neural Networks

Convolutional neural networks are among the most dominant deep learning methodologies since they are designated as techniques with a remarkable capacity for image analysis and classification. Their architecture is originated from the perceptron model in which a series of fully connected layers is established, and all neurons from consecutive layers are individually interconnected. A detailed description of all different types of layers follows.

Concerning the first layer in the architecture, the "convolutional" layer is named after the type of neural network. Its role is substantial for CNNs since this layer is responsible for the formation of activation maps. In particular, specific patterns of an image are extracted, helping the algorithm detect various characteristics essential for image classification [34,60]. Then, a pooling layer follows, whose duty is image downsampling, whereas any unwanted noise that might fuzzy the algorithm is appropriately discarded. This layer retains the set of pixel values that exceed a threshold optimally defined, rejecting all the remaining. For this process, the elements within a matrix that are in line with specific requirements concerning the maximum or average value are correctly selected.

The last part of a CNN architecture comprises one or more fully connected layers assigned for the "flattening" of the previous layer's output every time. This is considered as the final output layer, which takes the form of a vector. According to the values of the outcome vector, a specific label is assigned by the algorithm to every image. On the whole, the set of the fully connected layers are classified into distinct subcategories emanated from their role. For instance, the vectorization is attained by the first layer, whereas the category of each class given is defined by the final layer [61,62].

Concerning the activation function in the CNN models, the rectified linear unit (ReLU) is deployed in all convolutional and fully connected layers, while the sigmoid function serves as the final most common activation function in the output nodes [62]. It is worth mentioning that selecting the most suitable activation function is crucial and dependent on the desired outcome. The Softmax function can be efficiently utilized for the multiclass classification task. It has the ability to target class probabilities through a normalization process conducted on the actual output values derived from the last fully connected layer [62].

2.4. Methodology

This work discusses the recently proposed RGB-CNN model as a new efficient method in scintigraphy/ nuclear medical image analysis, regarding its application on the classification of SPECT MPI scans in coronary artery disease patients. This two-class classification task involves the cases of ischemia or infarction presence as well as those being labeled as normal in a sample of 224 patients. It particularly involves three distinctive processes, which are pre-processing, network design and testing/evaluation. These stages have been previously presented in common publications (see [30,50,53]). The pre-processing step consists of data normalization, data shuffle, data augmentation and data split into training, validation and testing. Data augmentation involves specific image processes such as range, enlargement, rotation and flip. The augmentation process is conducted before its entrance into the exploration and training of CNN. Concerning data split, the training dataset regards 85% of the provided dataset of 275 MPI images, whereas the remaining 15% is used for testing purposes. Next, the network design stage deals with the construction of a proper architecture through an exploration process. Then, the testing phase follows, utilizing the best CNN model derived. In the final stage, the produced CNN model is tested using unknown to the model data.

Likewise, the respective classification approach is deployed for the tasks of image pre-processing, network training and testing, and is applied to the new dataset. The process for the examined dataset of SPECT MPI scans is visually represented in Figure 2.

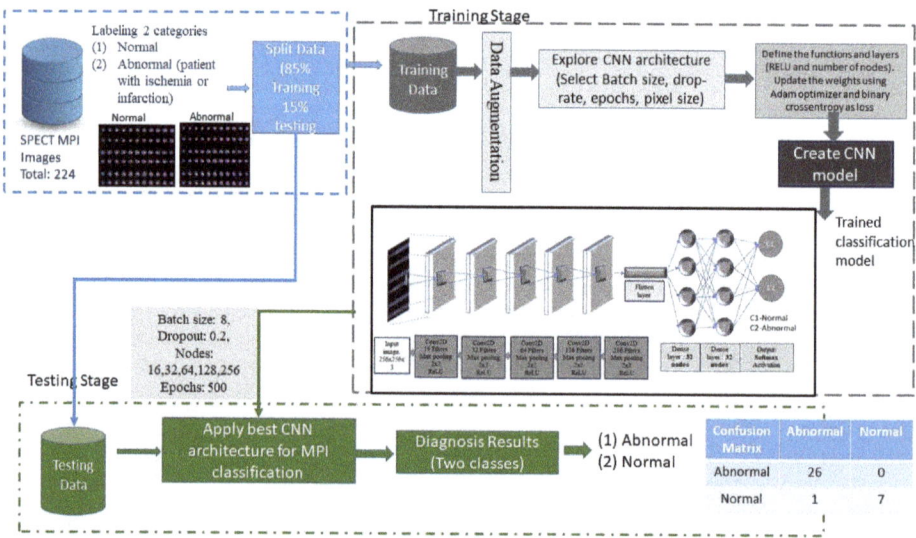

Figure 2. The proposed methodology for SPECT MPI classification including RGB-CNN architectures.

3. Methodology

3.1. RGB-Based CNN Architecture for Classification in Nuclear Medical Imaging

In this research study, we apply an efficient and robust CNN model, the RGB-CNN (proposed in a recent study in the domain of bone scintigraphy), to precisely categorize MPI images as normal or abnormal suffering from CAD. The developed CNN will demonstrate its capacity for high accuracy utilizing a fast yet straightforward architecture regarding MPI classification. A number of experiments were performed for different values of parameters, like pixels, epochs, drop rate, batch size, number of nodes and layers as described in [56–58]. Then, appropriate features are extracted and selected manually, following the most common classic feature extraction techniques. On the other hand, CNNs that resemble ANNs, achieve automatic feature extraction by applying multiple filters on the input images. Next, they proceed in selecting the most suitable for image classification through an advanced learning process.

A deep-layer network is constructed within this framework, embodying five convolutional-pooling layers, two dense layers, a dropout layer, followed by a final two-node output layer (see Figure 3).

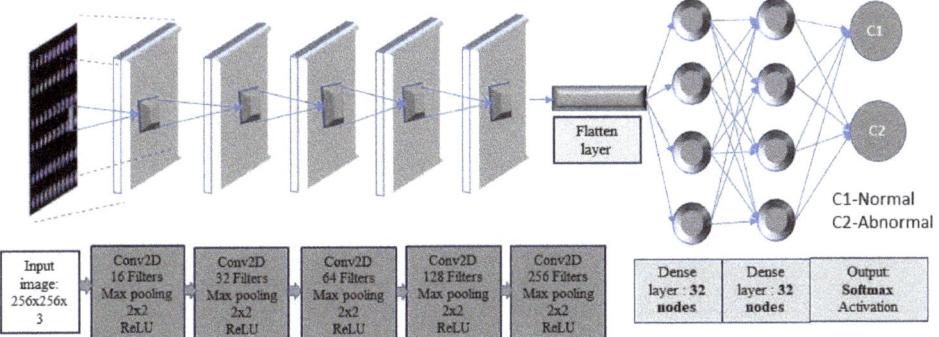

Figure 3. RGB-CNN architecture for CAD classification using SPECT MPI scans.

The dimensions of the input images vary from 250 × 250 pixels to 400 × 400 pixels. According to the structure of the proposed CNN, the initial convolutional layer includes 3 × 3 filters (kernels) followed by a 2 × 2-sized max-pooling layer and a dropout layer entailing a dropout rate of 0.2. The first convolutional layer is formed by 16 filters, whereas each layer that follows includes a double number of filters compared with the previous one. The same form is followed by the max-pooling layers that come next. A flattening operation is then utilized to transform the 2-dimension matrices to 1-dimension arrays so that they are inserted into the hidden dense layer of 64 nodes. The role of the dropout layer that follows is to randomly drop the learned weights by 20% to avoid overfitting. The output two-node layer comes as last in the proposed CNN model architecture.

The most common function utilized by CNNs is ReLU, which is applied to all convolutional and fully connected (dense) layers. In the output nodes, the categorical cross-entropy function is applied. The algorithm is tested through multiple runs by trying a different number of epochs varying from 200 to 700 to fully exploit the most valid number of epochs for CNN training. In this context, the ImageDataGenerator class from Keras is used, providing specific augmentation tasks over images, such as rotation, shifting, flipping and zoom. Finally, the categorical cross-entropy function is considered as a performance metric applied for the calculation of loss. It employs the ADAM optimizer, an adaptive learning rate optimization algorithm [36].

3.2. Deep Learning Models, Including Transfer Learning for CAD Classification in Medical Imaging

In this subsection, we introduce the process followed in this study on applying deep learning architectures, including transfer learning for benchmark CNN models in CAD diagnosis.

In deep learning model development, the traditional pipeline is the neural network training from scratch, which depends highly on the size of the data provided. Transfer learning is an alternative, most preferred and used process in developing deep learning architectures [63]. This process offers the capability to sufficiently employ the existing knowledge of a pre-trained CNN through the use of ImageNet dataset so as to result in competent predictions.

For an accurate classification process, an improved model training process is required, which derives from the incorporation of transfer learning during the training phase of the proposed CNN architectures. More specifically, the ImageNet [63,64] dataset needs to be utilized for network pre-training, thus resulting in accurate classification of medical SPECT myocardial perfusion imaging scans into two categories, namely normal and abnormal (patient with ischemia or infarction). According to the relevant literature, the ImageNet dataset is employed by the popular CNN methods for model pre-training and includes 1.4 million images with 1000 classes. Based on this pre-training process, VGG16 and DenseNet models are trained to extract particular features from images through the assignment of constant weights on them. The number of the weight layers affects the depth of the model, along with the steps needed for feature extraction.

The training dataset, representing 85% of the provided dataset of 224 SPECT MPI images, is loaded into the pre-trained models after undergoing a proper augmentation process. Hence, an improved CNN model is produced, which is inserted into the next testing phase. The remaining 15% of the provided dataset is accordingly incorporated into the evaluation process. The proposed transfer learning methodology of the state-of-the-art CNN models is graphically presented in Figure 4, regarding the examined dataset of 224 patients.

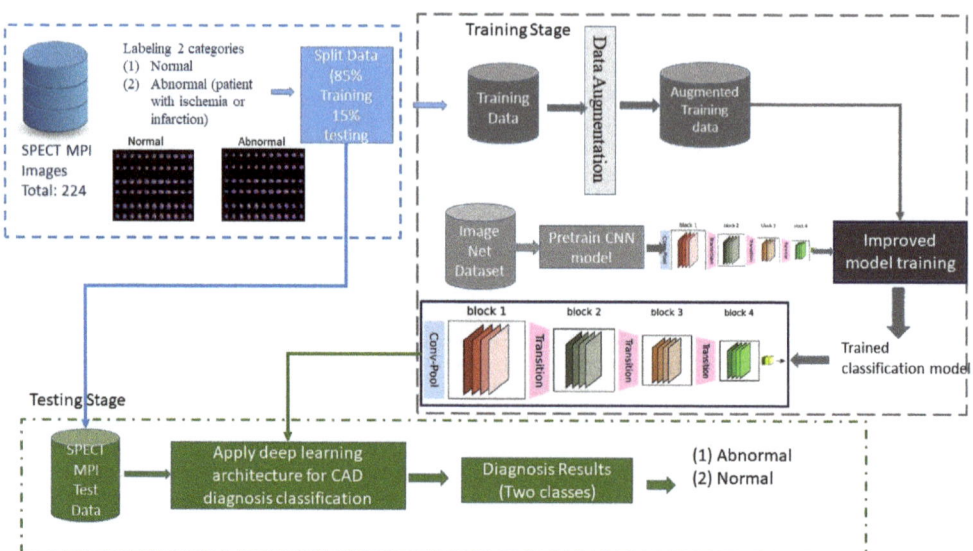

Figure 4. The proposed methodology for SPECT MPI classification including RGB-CNN architectures.

Following the process in which the benchmark CNN model is selected for the classification task, the exploration and identification of suitable, robust and efficient architectures of these CNN models come next for the specific problem solving, which concerns the identification of the correct category of CAD diagnosis. On this basis, the fine-tuning of the model parameters and the configuration of several other hyperparameters were successfully attained through a thorough investigation regarding the appropriate deep learning architecture. For comparison purposes, various common deep learning architectures such as Densenet, VGG16, Mobilienet and InceptionV3 were investigated.

4. Results

This study attempts to address this image classification problem considering the classification of images into 2 categories: normal and abnormal (ischemic or infarction patient cases). The classification processes were individually repeated 10 times to produce the overall classification accuracy.

All the simulations were performed in Google Colab [65], a cloud-based environment that supports free GPU acceleration. The Keras 2.0.2 and TensorFlow 2.0.0 frameworks were utilized to develop the employed deep learning architectures. Image augmentations (like rotations, shifting, zoom, flips and more) took place only during the training process of the deep networks and were accomplished using the ImageDataGenerator class from Keras. The investigated deep learning architectures were coded in the Python programming language. Sci-Kit Learn was used for data normalization, data splitting, calculation of confusion matrices and classification reports. It should be noted that all images produced by the scanning device and used as the dataset in this research were in RGB format, providing 3-channel color information.

4.1. Results from RGB-CNN

In this study, a meticulous CNN exploration process regarding the deep learning architectures of RGB-CNN was accomplished. In particular, an experimental analysis was conducted, where various drop rates (between 0.1–0.9), epochs (200 to 700), number of dense nodes (like 16–16, 32–32, 64–64, 128–128, 256–256, 512–512 and 1024–1024), pixel sizes (from 200 × 200 × 3 up to 450 × 450 × 3) and batch sizes (8, 16, 32 and 64) were tested. To prevent overfitting [62] in the proposed deep learning architectures, the authors conducted an exploratory analysis for different dropouts and numbers of epochs. According to the conducted analysis results, a dropout value of 0.2 and the set of 500 epochs were adequate to produce satisfactory results for the investigated RGB-CNN architecture.

Moreover, an exploration analysis involving the testing of various pixel sizes was conducted. The best pixel size of the input images was determined as regards the classification accuracy and loss. Figures 5 and 6 illustrate the produced results in terms of accuracy for the examined pixel sizes, for both CNN-based architectures. These figures foster the successful selection of the appropriate pixel size for each architecture which is 250 × 250 × 3 for RGB-CNN.

Following this exploration process, several configurations, including dropout = 0.2 and three batch sizes (8, 16 and 32), various pixel sizes and dense nodes in RGB-CNN model consisting of 5 layers (16–32–64–128–256) were investigated. Tables 1–3 illustrate the results produced for the relevant pixel sizes for the well-performed batch sizes of 8, 16 and 32. These results helped in the selection of the most appropriate pixel size, which is 250 × 250 × 3.

As regards the two dense blocks that are the last ones in both architectures, a rigorous exploration process was performed to determine the best configuration in terms of accuracy (validation and testing) and loss. The results are depicted in Figures 3 and 4 regarding 4 and 5 convolutional layers, respectively. Looking at the specific figures, it emerges that 64–64 is the optimum combination for the CNN model.

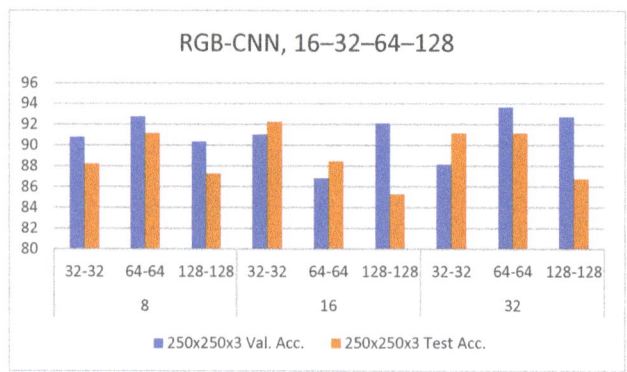

Figure 5. RGB-CNN architecture with 4 layers, various dense nodes and batch sizes for CAD classification problem.

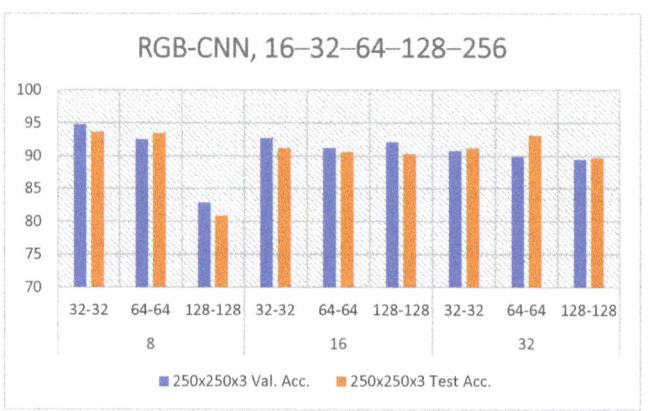

Figure 6. RGB-CNN architecture with 5 layers, various dense nodes and batch sizes for CAD classification problem.

Table 1. Results for various pixel sizes and dense nodes in RGB-CNN with 5 layers (16–32–64–128–256), dropout = 0.2 and batch size = 8.

Pixels	Dense Nodes	Val. Acc.	Val. Loss	Test Acc.	Test Loss	AUC	Time (s)
200 × 200 × 3	32–32	90.12	0.25	89.7	0.31	0.916	890
	64–64	93.41	0.2	92.64	0.21	0.935	831
	128–128	89.05	0.36	89.21	0.33	0.871	860
250 × 250 × 3	32–32	**94.72**	**0.16**	**93.62**	**0.12**	**0.926**	1125
	64–64	92.53	0.25	93.47	0.13	0.921	1116
	128–128	82.89	0.44	80.87	0.18	0.845	1043
300 × 300 × 3	32–32	90.78	0.17	88.23	0.28	0.9025	1736
	64–64	85.3	0.36	86.47	0.29	0.893	1641
	128–128	86.84	0.45	73.52	0.69	0.716	1469
350 × 350 × 3	32–32	78.94	0.51	70.58	0.61	0.78	2200
	64–64	80.52	0.47	68.35	0.62	0.765	2221
	128–128	74.21	0.57	65.43	0.71	0.711	2185

Table 2. Results for various pixel sizes and dense nodes in RGB-CNN with 5 layers (16–32–64–128–256). dropout = 0.2 and batch size = 16.

Pixels	Dense Nodes	Val. Acc.	Val. Loss	Test Acc.	Test Loss	AUC	Time (s)
200 × 200 × 3	32–32	92.73	0.183	92.15	0.24	0.885	748
	64–64	92.53	0.24	93.13	0.265	0.948	679
	128–128	91.72	0.23	89.91	0.22	0.885	674
250 × 250 × 3	32–32	94.73	0.12	91.17	0.22	0.769	990
	64–64	91.21	0.235	90.36	0.26	0.873	971
	128–128	92.1	0.195	90.3	0.21	0.898	1089
300 × 300 × 3	32–32	94.73	0.158	91.66	0.21	0.920	1547
	64–64	91.42	0.24	91.905	0.183	0.93	1387
	128–128	92.03	0.19	92.01	0.218	0.915	1409
350 × 350 × 3	32–32	88.46	0.31	87.74	0.29	0.871	1854
	64–64	89.47	0.325	91.17	0.198	0.887	1856
	128–128	92.1	0.185	92.01	0.205	0.914	1910

Table 3. Results for various pixel sizes and dense nodes in RGB-CNN with 5 layers (16–32–64–128–256). dropout = 0.2 and batch size = 32.

Pixels	Dense Nodes	Val. Acc.	Val. Loss	Test Acc.	Test Loss	AUC	Time (s)
200 × 200 × 3	32–32	87.71	0.323	92.15	0.31	0.935	630
	64–64	90.34	0.33	91.9	0.3	0.931	790
	128–128	93.82	0.18	92.04	0.245	0.923	707
250 × 250 × 3	32–32	90.78	0.2	91.17	0.21	0.855	1110
	64–64	89.91	0.253	93.12	0.187	0.921	1065
	128–128	89.47	0.263	89.69	0.305	0.909	1039
300 × 300 × 3	32–32	88.59	0.29	90.19	0.276	0.917	1440
	64–64	89.46	0.224	91.15	0.24	0.907	1569
	128–128	92.1	0.21	91.37	0.2	0.914	1573
350 × 350 × 3	32–32	87.28	0.26	88.57	0.23	0.898	1650
	64–64	90.78	0.38	86.77	0.42	0.854	2077
	128–128	89.47	0.295	91.17	0.245	0.898	1980

Next, for the selected pixel size (250 × 250 × 3), different batch sizes (8, 16 and 32) with various configurations in dense nodes were investigated, also utilizing the two previously best-performed architectures concerning the number of convolutional layers (which are 16–32–64–128 and 16–32–64–128–256), as presented in recent research studies [56–58]. The outcomes of this exploration are presented in Figures 5 and 6. These figures show that the best CNN configuration corresponds to batch size 8, five convolutional layers (16–32–64–128–256) and dense nodes 32–32. It emerges that dense 32–32 is the most suitable configuration concerning the dense nodes.

Figure 7 shows the accuracy, loss and AUC values for various dense nodes regarding the best batch size (8) and the number of convolutional layers (16–32–64–128–256).

Additionally, further exploration analysis was performed for various numbers of convolutional layers. Some indicative results are presented in Figure 8. It is observed that the model was able to increase its classification accuracy for 5 convolutional layers significantly.

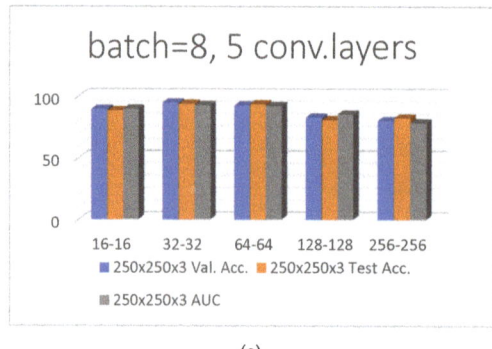
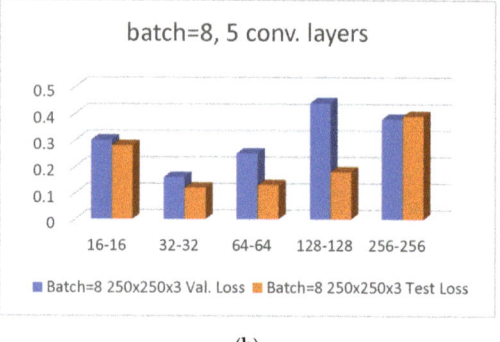

Figure 7. Results for the best RGB-CNN configuration concerning (**a**) accuracy and AUC score and (**b**) loss.

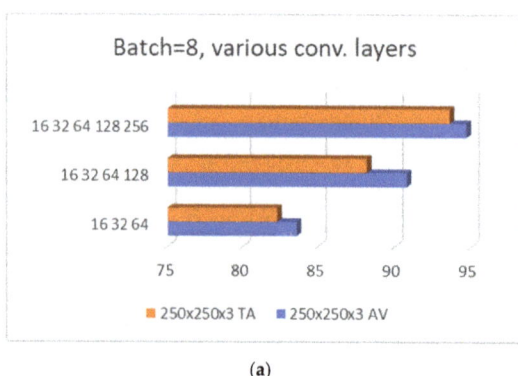
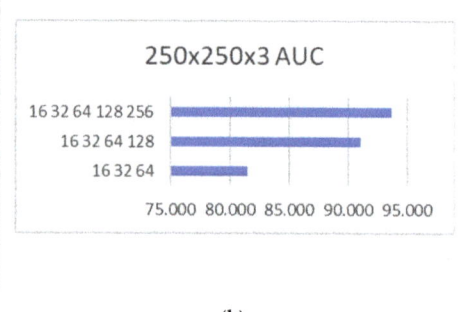

Figure 8. CNN results for different numbers of convolutional layers concerning (**a**) validation and testing accuracies and (**b**) AUC values.

To sum-up, the best RGB-CNN architecture with this problem is: pixel size (250 × 250 × 3), batch size = 8, dropout = 0.2, conv 16–32–64–128–256, dense nodes 32.32, epochs = 500 (average run time = 1125 s).

In addition, Table 4 depicts the confusion matrix of the best VGG16 architecture. Figure 9 illustrates the classification accuracies (validation and testing) with their respective loss curves for the proposed RGB-CNN architecture. Figure 10 depicts the diagnostic performance of RGB-CNN model in SPECT MPI interpretation assessed by ROC analysis for CAD patients.

In the proposed method, the early stopping condition for RGB-CNN was investigated considering 100 epochs, thus providing adequate accuracy, higher than that of the other CNNs. In particular, the produced accuracy for early stopping was approximately 89% in most of the examined runs. However, using the minimum error stopping condition, the capacity of the algorithm was explored, increasing the accuracy of the RGB-CNN model up to 94% approximately. Figure 9a illustrates the precision curves presenting a smooth change in accuracy for the proposed model.

Table 4. Best confusion matrix for the proposed RGB-CNN.

2-Classes	Abnormal	Normal
Abnormal	26	0
Normal	1	7

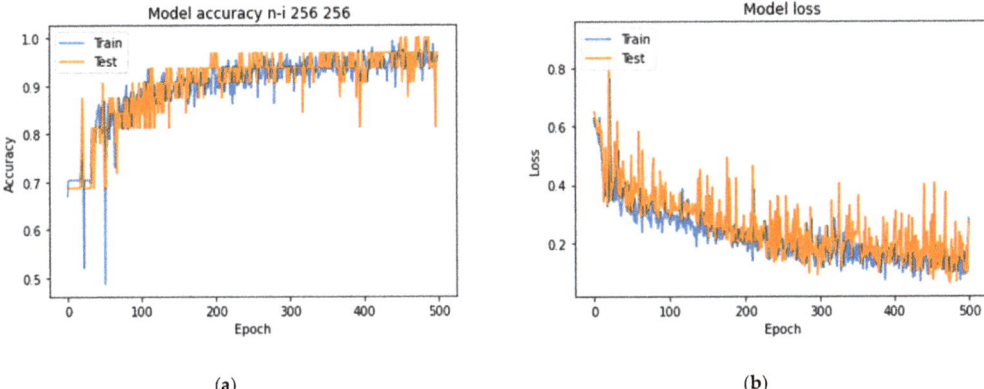

Figure 9. Precision curves for best RGB-CNN model showing (a) accuracy and (b) loss.

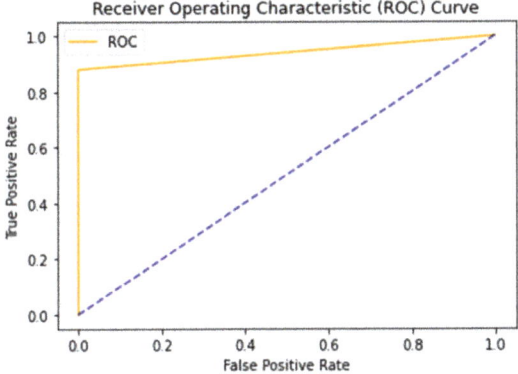

Figure 10. Diagnostic performance of RGB-CNN model in SPECT MPI interpretation assessed by ROC analysis for CAD patients. ROC = receiver operating characteristic, AUC = area under the curve, PPV = positive predictive value, NPV = negative predictive value.

4.2. Results from Deep Learning Architectures Applying Transfer Learning and Comparative Analysis

In this subsection, the second deep learning classification approach of CAD patients using transfer learning was implemented, followed by a comparative analysis. Following the process discussed in Section 2.4, transfer learning was utilized employing several pretrained CNN models, avoiding training a new network with randomly initialized weights. In this way, the classification process of SPECT MPI scans is faster and more efficient due to the limited number of training images.

This approach includes efficient state-of-the-art CNNs in the medical image analysis domain, which were mainly reported in previous studies in similar classification tasks. In particular, for the purpose of this research work, certain SoA CNN architectures such as: (i) VGG16 [39], (ii) DenseNet in [43], (iii) MobileNet [59], and (iv) Inception V3 [60] were used.

Concerning the training characteristics of this approach, the stochastic gradient descent with momentum algorithm was used, and the initial learning rate was set to 0.0001. It is worth mentioning that an exploratory analysis for the SoA CNNs [25,33] was previously conducted in the reported literature, paying particular attention to overfitting avoidance [62]. Overfitting is a common issue in most state-of-the-art CNNs that work with small datasets; thus, a meticulous exploration with various dropout, dense layers and batch sizes was applied to avoid it. Overall, the CNN selection and optimization of the hyperparameters was performed following an exploration process considering a combination of values for batch-size (8, 16, 32, 64, and 128), dropout (0.2, 0.5, 0.7 and 0.9), flatten layer, number of trainable layers and various pixel sizes (200 × 200 × 3 up to 350 × 350 × 3). Moreover, a divergent number of dense nodes, like 16, 32, 64, 128, 256 and 512 was explored. The number of epochs ranged from 200 up to 500. The best-performing CNN models in terms of accuracy and loss function in the validation phase were selected as the optimum for classifying the test dataset [24,56].

After the extensive exploration of all the provided architectures of popular CNNs, the authors defined the optimum values for the respective models' parameters, as follows:

- VGG16: pixel size (300 × 300 × 3), batch size = 32, dropout = 0.2, Global Average Poolong2D, dense nodes 64 × 64, epochs = 400, (average run time = 1853 s),
- DenseNet: pixel size (250 × 250 × 3), batch size = 8, dropout = 0.2, Global Average Poolong2D, dense nodes 16 × 16, epochs = 400, (average run time = 2074 s),
- MobileNet: pixel size (250 × 250 × 3), batch size = 8, dropout = 0.2, Global Average Poolong2D, dense nodes 32 × 32, epochs = 400, (average run time = 3070 s),
- InceptionV3: pixel size (300 × 300 × 3), batch size = 8, dropout = 0.2, Global Average Poolong2D, dense nodes 256 × 256, epochs = 400, (average run time = 1538 s).

Concerning the dropout value, 0.2 was selected as the best-performed for the investigated CNN configurations, according to the exploration process. The testing image dataset was used to evaluate the network's performance; however it is not involved in the training phase.

The results of the explored SoA CNN architectures proposed in the second approach are compared to the best-performed RGB-CNN model. They are gathered in the following three figures. More specifically, Figure 11 depicts the classification accuracy in validation and testing phases for the best-performed deep learning architectures. Figure 12 illustrates the respective loss for all SoA CNNs. Finally, Figure 13 presents the AUC score values for all performed CNNs.

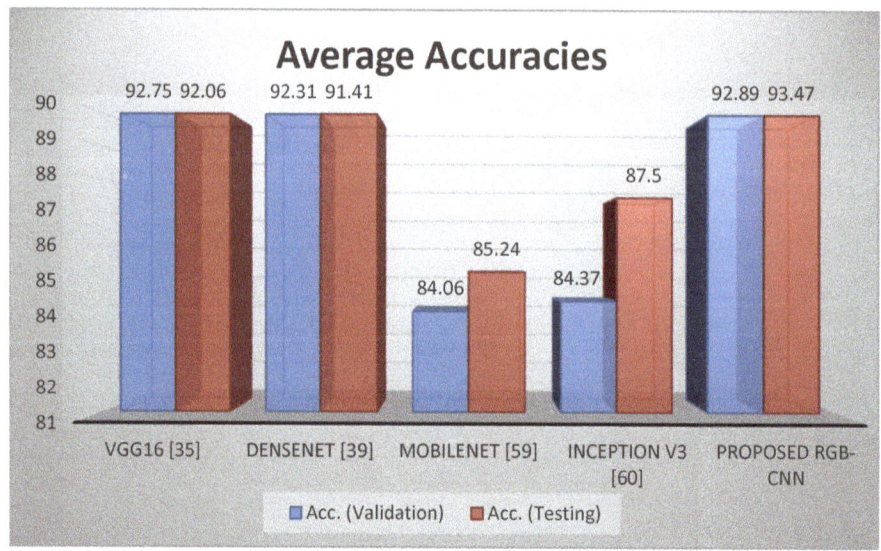

Figure 11. Comparison of the classification accuracies for all performed CNNs.

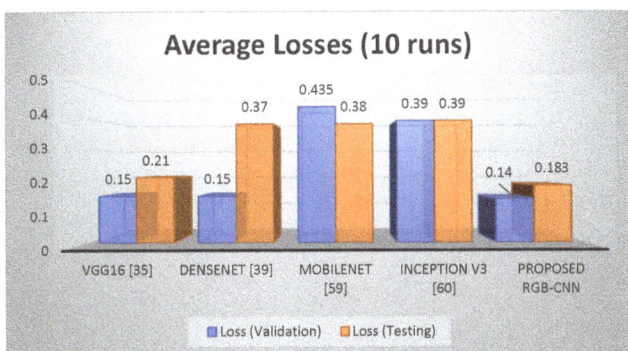

Figure 12. Comparison of loss (validation and testing) for all performed CNNs.

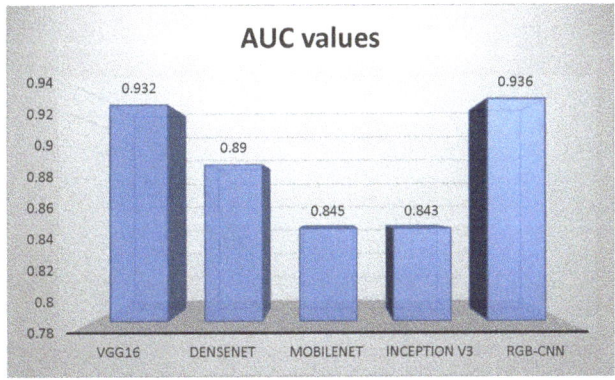

Figure 13. AUC score values for all performed CNNs.

5. Discussion of Results and Conclusions

Due to their ability to track complex visual patterns, powerful and widely used CNN algorithms are employed in the medical image analysis domain to address the problem of CAD diagnosis in nuclear cardiology. In this research study, two different deep learning classification approaches, namely, the RGB-based CNN model and the transfer learning-based CNN models (the benchmark CNN models pre-trained by ImageNet dataset), were adopted to identify perfusion defects through the use of SPECT MPI scans. The first classification approach is based on RGB-CNN algorithms, previously proposed for image classification in nuclear medicine regarding bone scintigraphy. The second approach utilizes transfer learning incorporated in well-known deep learning architectures. The provided dataset, comprising stress and rest images from 224 subjects, is employed to assess the proposed models with respect to their performance. The problem was formulated as a two-class classification problem.

For an in-depth assessment of the results, a comparative analysis regarding the classification performance of the proposed model against that of other CNNs reported in the literature is performed (even indirectly) in the examined field of CAD diagnosis in nuclear medicine, using solely SPECT-MPI images. A decent amount of relevant research studies in this scientific field was gathered in Introduction and presented in Table 5, followed by the classification accuracies and evaluation metrics of the respective models. As regards the previous works of [50–52], where polar map images were used for CAD classification, deep CNNs and graph-based CNNs were employed for normal/abnormal classification. These are not related to this research study and provide classification accuracies up to 91%.

Table 5. Related works in coronary artery disease classification using ML and DL techniques.

Reference	Input Data	ML/DL Methods	Classification Problem	Reference Standard	Results
			Quantitative Data and Clinical Data from Polar Maps		
Arsanjani et al. [48]	Quantitative data	Boosted ensemble learning	Normal/Abnormal	Coronary Angiography	Stress TPD: Accuracy 0.88, AUC 0.94, Specificity 0.93, Sensitivity 0.81
Hu et al. [45], 2020	Clinical and quantitative data	Ensemble LogitBoost algorithm (ML)	Normal/Abnormal	Coronary Angiography	Accuracy 0.72, AUC 0.79.
Rahmani et al. [47], 2019	Clinical and Quantitative data	Feed-forward ANN (multi-layer perceptron)	Absence/Presence of coronary artery stenosis >50% in at least a vessel	Coronary Angiography	Accuracy 0.86, Specificity 1.00, Sensitivity 0.82
		Feed-forward ANN	(2 classes) Normal/Abnormal angiography result	Coronary Angiography	Accuracy 0.93, Specificity 1.00, Sensitivity 0.92
Arsanjani et al. [55]	Quantitative and functional data	SVM	Absence/Presence of coronary artery stenosis ≥70%	Coronary Angiography	Stress TPD: Accuracy 0.86, AUC 0.92, Specificity 0.88, Sensitivity 0.84
Guner et al. [49], 2010	Quantitative polar maps	ANN: multilayer perceptron (WEKA), input layer of 50 nodes, one hidden layer of 5 nodes and one output node.	Absence/Presence of coronary artery stenosis	Coronary Angiography	AUC 0.74, Specificity 0.68, Sensitivity 0.71

Table 5. *Cont.*

Reference	Input Data	ML/DL Methods	Classification Problem	Reference Standard	Results
		Polar Maps (Images)			
Betancur et al. [50], 2019	Upright and supine polar maps	DL: 3 × (Conv.Layers, Relu, Max-Pooling filter) and 3 fully connected layers.	Presence of coronary artery stenosis ≥70% and >50% in left main coronary artery (Normal/Abnormal)	Coronary Angiography	The AUC score, specificity and sensitivity were 81%, 83%, and 66%
Betancur et al. [51], 2018	Raw and quantitative polar maps	Deep CNN: 3 × (Conv.Layers, Relu, Max-Pooling filter), 3 fully connected layers, followed by 3 parallel outputs—1 per coronary territory	Presence of coronary artery stenosis ≥70% (Normal/Abnormal)	Coronary Angiography	The AUC score, specificity and sensitivity were 80%, 58%, and 82%
Spier et al. [52], 2019	Polar maps	Graph-based CNN, Chebyshev	Presence of coronary artery stenosis (Normal/Abnormal)	Expert Reader	The accuracy, specificity and sensitivity were 91%, 96%, and 86%
		2D SPECT MPI images			
Berkaya et al. [53], 2020	SPECT MPI images	SVM with deep features, VGG-19	(2 classes) Normal, Abnormal	Expert Reader	The accuracy, specificity and sensitivity were 79%, 57%, and 100%
		SVM with shallow features, VGG-19	(2 classes) Normal, Abnormal	Expert Reader	The accuracy, specificity and sensitivity were 94%, 100%, and 88%
		Transfer learning, VGG-16	(2 classes) Normal, Abnormal	Expert Reader	The accuracy, AUC, specificity and sensitivity were 86%, 92%, 71%, and 100%
		Knowledge-based	(2 classes) Normal, Abnormal	Expert Reader	The accuracy, specificity and sensitivity were 93%, 86%, and 100%
Proposed work	SPECT MPI images	RGB-CNN batch size = 8, dropout = 0.2, conv 16-32-64-128-256, dense nodes 32.32	(2 classes) Normal, Abnormal	Coronary Angiography	The accuracy, AUC, specificity and sensitivity were 94%, 93%, 78%, and 94%

It is worth mentioning that only one previous work is highly related to the current research study and regards the presence of coronary artery stenosis (normal or abnormal) as a two-class classification problem. This work employed well-known CNNs to classify normal/abnormal patient cases [53], utilizing transfer learning. The authors employ deep neural networks that underwent a pre-training phase as well as an SVM classifier characterized by deep and shallow features derived from the respective networks. Most of the applied DL-based methods (AlexNet, GoogleNet, DenseNet, Resnet, VGG-16) in this dataset provided accuracies less than 87%, and only the VGG-19 utilizing SVM with shallow features increased the accuracy slightly. The knowledge-based classification model, which uses extracted features based on shapes and empirically verified parameters, fine-tuned on the training and validation images, provided the highest classification accuracy of up to 93%. Through the conducted comparative analysis of the proposed RGB-CNN method with the related ML and deep learning techniques as listed in Table 5, it is concluded that the proposed RGB-CNN model outperforms all the previous techniques in MPI imaging. It provides slightly better performance in classification accuracy (94%) and AUC score (93%), making it a competitive solution to this diagnosis task.

Following the process of rigorously exploring possible hyperparameters and regularization methods of the proposed RGB-CNN architecture, the best overall classification accuracy for the deep network model (best RGB-CNN) was established (see Figures 11–13). Authors selected the RGB-CNN model with 5 convolutional layers, batch size = 16, dropout = 0.2 and 64–64 dense nodes as the simplest and most optimum performed CNN, concerning testing accuracy and loss. Moreover, from the results above, it appears that the best RGB-CNN model is characterized by an overall classification accuracy of 93.47% $\pm$ 2.81% when the produced overall test loss is approximately 0.18 (see Figure 12). To lay emphasis on the classification performance of the CNN approaches presented in this study, the authors followed a comparative analysis between the proposed RGB-CNN model and other SoA CNNs, commonly used for image classification problems, with reference to accuracy and other metrics such as the AUC score. Regarding the produced AUC value for the RGB-CNN models and the other SoA CNNs, as depicted in Figure 13, RGB-CNN seems to have the highest AUC score, making it possibly the best classifier in terms of performance for the given problem. The average run time of the best architecture for the proposed model is 1125 s which is considered fast for such types of networks. Similar to the other CNN-based methods, this method presents faster run time as shown in the previous works of the same team of authors [33,56] in the case of bone scintigraphy.

The results indicate that the proposed RGB-CNN is an efficient, robust and straightforward deep neural network able to detect perfusion abnormalities related to myocardial ischemia and infarction on SPECT images in nuclear medicine image analysis. It was also demonstrated that this is a model of low complexity and generalization capabilities compared to the state-of-the-art deep neural networks. Moreover, it exhibits better performance than the SoA CNN architectures applied in the specific problem regarding accuracy and AUC values. The proposed CNN-based classification approach can be employed in the case of SPECT-MPI scans in nuclear cardiology and can support CAD diagnosis. It can as well contribute as a clinical decision support system in nuclear medicine imaging.

To sum up, among the major differences of RGB-CNN compared to other conventional CNNs are (i) their ability to efficiently train a model considering a small dataset without the need to undergo network pre-training with ImageNet dataset, (ii) their ability to be optimized through an exploratory analysis which helps to avoid overfitting and generalize well to unknown input images, and (iii) their less complex architecture which enhances their performance in an efficient run time [33,57].

Regarding the limitations presented in previous studies, the models proposed in this work do not depend on specific characteristics like gender and camera specifications that can elevate the number of inputs [34]. In addition, they can perform sufficiently, even when not many training images are available. Among the privileges the proposed models enjoy is their ability to use SPECT images as input without the need for any additional data. This feature is rather distinguishing between this work and other studies. Finally, less experienced physicians can improve their diagnostic accuracy by supporting their opinion with the results of such systems. However, there are some limitations that need to be considered in future work. These are (i) the limited number of normal cases in the dataset, making it unbalanced, and (ii) the disregard of clinical and other functional data in the classification process, which would improve the diagnosis.

According to the overall results of this study, the proposed deep learning structures of RGB-CNN are accredited for being extremely efficient in classifying SPECT MPI scans in nuclear medicine. Even though these effective CNN-based approaches use a relatively limited number of patients, this study further considers a deep learning classification methodology, incorporating transfer learning, and in collaboration with the well-known CNN models, as a technique that can have a considerable impact on myocardial perfusion detection.

As a typical black box AI-based method, deep learning lacks clarity and reasoning for the decision, which is highly important in medical diagnosis. Since DL models are often criticized because of their internal unclear decision-making process, explainable AI systems should come with causal models of the world supporting explanation and understanding. Recent research efforts are directed towards developing more interpretable models, focusing on the understandability of the DL-based methods.

Future work is also oriented toward the acquisition of more scan images of patients suffering from CAD, with a view to expand the current research and validate the efficacy of the proposed architecture. But, overall, the findings of this work seem highly reassuring, particularly when the computer-aided diagnosis is involved, establishing the proposed CNN-based models as a suitable tool in everyday clinical work.

Author Contributions: Conceptualization, N.P.; methodology, E.P. and N.P.; software, E.P.; validation, N.P., E.P.; formal analysis, N.P. and E.P.; investigation, E.P. and N.P.; resources, N.P.; data curation, N.P.; writing—original draft preparation, N.P.; writing—review and editing, E.P., N.P.; visualization, E.P.; supervision, N.P. and E.P. All authors have read and agreed to the published version of the manuscript.

Funding: This research received no external funding.

Institutional Review Board Statement: This research work does not report human experimentation; not involve human participants following an experimentation in subjects. All procedures in this study were in accordance with the Declaration of Helsinki.

Informed Consent Statement: This study was approved by the Board Committee Director of the Diagnostic Medical Center "Diagnostiko-Iatriki A.E." Vasilios Parafestas and the requirement to obtain informed consent was waived by the Director of the Diagnostic Center due to its retrospective nature.

Data Availability Statement: The datasets analyzed during the current study are available from the nuclear medicine physician on reasonable request.

Conflicts of Interest: The authors declare no conflict of interest.

References

1. Cassar, A.; Holmes, D.R.; Rihal, C.S.; Gersh, B.J. Chronic Coronary Artery Disease: Diagnosis and Management. *Mayo Clin. Proc.* **2009**, *84*, 1130–1146. [CrossRef]
2. Ross, R. Atherosclerosis—An Inflammatory Disease. *N. Engl. J. Med.* **1999**, *340*, 115–126. [CrossRef]
3. Girelli, M.; Martinelli, N.; Peyvandi, F.; Olivieri, O. Genetic Architecture of Coronary Artery Disease in the Genome-Wide Era: Implications for the Emerging "Golden Dozen" Loci. *Semin. Thromb. Hemost.* **2009**, *35*, 671–682. [CrossRef]
4. Álvarez-Álvarez, M.M.; Zanetti, D.; Carreras-Torres, R.; Moral, P.; Athanasiadis, G. A survey of sub-Saharan gene flow into the Mediterranean at risk loci for coronary artery disease. *Eur. J. Hum. Genet.* **2017**, *25*, 472–476. [CrossRef] [PubMed]
5. Łukaszewski, B.; Nazar, J.; Goch, M.; Łukaszewska, M.; Stępiński, A.; Jurczyk, M. Diagnostic methods for detection of bone metastases. *Współczesna Onkol.* **2017**, *21*, 98–103. [CrossRef] [PubMed]
6. Sartor, O. Radium and targeted alpha therapy in prostate cancer: New data and concepts. *Ann. Oncol.* **2020**, *31*, 165–166. [CrossRef] [PubMed]

7. Underwood, S.R.; Anagnostopoulos, C.; Cerqueira, M.; Ell, P.J.; Flint, E.J.; Harbinson, M.; Kelion, A.D.; Al-Mohammad, A.; Prvulovich, E.M.; Shaw, L.J.; et al. Myocardial perfusion scintigraphy: The evidence. *Eur. J. Nucl. Med. Mol. Imaging* **2004**, *31*, 261–291. [CrossRef] [PubMed]
8. Schuijf, J.D.; Poldermans, D.; Shaw, L.J.; Jukema, J.W.; Lamb, H.J.; De Roos, A.; Wijns, W.; Van Der Wall, E.E.; Bax, J.J. Diagnostic and prognostic value of non-invasive imaging in known or suspected coronary artery disease. *Eur. J. Nucl. Med. Mol. Imaging* **2005**, *33*, 93–104. [CrossRef]
9. Talbot, J.N.; Paycha, F.; Balogova, S. Diagnosis of bone metastasis: Recent comparative studies of imaging modalities. *Q. J. Nucl. Med. Mol. Imaging* **2011**, *55*, 374–410. [PubMed]
10. Doi, K. Computer-Aided Diagnosis in Medical Imaging: Historical Review, Current Status and Future Poten-tial. *Computerized medical imaging and graphics. Off. J. Comput. Med. Imaging Soc.* **2007**, *31*, 198–211. [CrossRef] [PubMed]
11. O'Sullivan, G.J.; Carty, F.L.; Cronin, C.G. Imaging of Bone Metastasis: An Update. *World J. Radiol.* **2015**, *7*, 202–211. [CrossRef]
12. Chang, C.Y.; Gill, C.M.; Simeone, F.J.; Taneja, A.K.; Huang, A.J.; Torriani, M.; A Bredella, M. Comparison of the diagnostic accuracy of 99 m-Tc-MDP bone scintigraphy and 18 F-FDG PET/CT for the detection of skeletal metastases. *Acta Radiol.* **2016**, *57*, 58–65. [CrossRef]
13. Wyngaert, T.V.D.; On behalf of the EANM Bone & Joint Committee and the Oncology Committee; Strobel, K.; Kampen, W.U.; Kuwert, T.; Van Der Bruggen, W.; Mohan, H.K.; Gnanasegaran, G.; Bolton, R.D.; Weber, W.A.; et al. The EANM practice guidelines for bone scintigraphy. *Eur. J. Nucl. Med. Mol. Imaging* **2016**, *43*, 1723–1738. [CrossRef]
14. Coleman, R. Metastatic bone disease: Clinical features, pathophysiology and treatment strategies. *Cancer Treat. Rev.* **2001**, *27*, 165–176. [CrossRef]
15. Savvopoulos, C.A.; Spyridonidis, T.; Papandrianos, N.; Vassilakos, P.J.; Alexopoulos, D.; Apostolopoulos, D.J. CT-based attenuation correction in Tl-201 myocardial perfusion scintigraphy is less effective than non-corrected SPECT for risk stratification. *J. Nucl. Cardiol.* **2014**, *21*, 519–531. [CrossRef]
16. Malek, H. Nuclear Cardiology. In *Practical Cardiology*; Elsevier BV: Amsterdam, The Netherlands, 2018; pp. 167–172.
17. American Heart Association Editorial Staff. Myocardial Perfusion Imaging (MPI) Test. Available online: https://www.heart.org/en/health-topics/heart-attack/diagnosing-a-heart-attack/myocardial-perfusion-imaging-mpi-test (accessed on 15 March 2021).
18. Alexanderson, E.; Better, N.; Bouyoucef, S.-E.; Dondi, M.; Dorbala, S.; Einstein, A.J.; El-Haj, N.; Giubbini, R.; Keng, F.; Kumar, A.; et al. *Nuclear Cardiology: Guidance on the Implementation of SPECT Myocardial Perfusion Imaging*; Human Health Series; International Atomic Energy Agency: Vienna, Australia, 2016.
19. Slart, R.H.J.A.; Williams, M.C.; Juarez-Orozco, L.E.; Rischpler, C.; Dweck, M.R.; Glaudemans, A.W.J.M.; Gimelli, A.; Georgoulias, P.; Gheysens, O.; Gaemperli, O.; et al. Position paper of the EACVI and EANM on artificial intelligence applications in multimodality cardiovascular imaging using SPECT/CT, PET/CT, and cardiac CT. *Eur. J. Nucl. Med. Mol. Imaging* **2021**, *48*, 1399–1413. [CrossRef] [PubMed]
20. Sartor, A.O.; DiBiase, S.J. Bone Metastases in Advanced Prostate Cancer: Management. 2018. Available online: https://www.uptodate.com/contents/bone-metastases-in-advanced-prostate-cancer-management (accessed on 7 July 2021).
21. Johansson, L.; Edenbrandt, L.; Nakajima, K.; Lomsky, M.; Svensson, S.-E.; Trägårdh, E. Computer-aided diagnosis system outperforms scoring analysis in myocardial perfusion imaging. *J. Nucl. Cardiol.* **2014**, *21*, 416–423. [CrossRef] [PubMed]
22. Slomka, P.J.; Betancur, J.; Liang, J.X.; Otaki, Y.; Hu, L.-H.; Sharir, T.; Dorbala, S.; Di Carli, M.; Fish, M.B.; Ruddy, T.D.; et al. Rationale and design of the REgistry of Fast Myocardial Perfusion Imaging with NExt generation SPECT (REFINE SPECT). *J. Nucl. Cardiol.* **2018**, *27*, 1010–1021. [CrossRef] [PubMed]
23. Juarez-Orozco, L.E.; Martinez-Manzanera, O.; Storti, A.E.; Knuuti, J. Machine Learning in the Evaluation of Myocardial Ischemia Through Nuclear Cardiology. *Curr. Cardiovasc. Imaging Rep.* **2019**, *12*, 5. [CrossRef]
24. Litjens, G.; Kooi, T.; Bejnordi, B.E.; Setio, A.A.A.; Ciompi, F.; Ghafoorian, M.; van der Laak, J.A.; van Ginneken, B.; Sánchez, C.I. A survey on deep learning in medical image analysis. *Med. Image Anal.* **2017**, *42*, 60–88. [CrossRef]
25. Suri, J.S. State-of-the-art review on deep learning in medical imaging. *Front. Biosci.* **2019**, *24*, 392–426. [CrossRef]
26. Lundervold, A.; Lundervold, A. An overview of deep learning in medical imaging focusing on MRI. *Z. Med. Phys.* **2019**, *29*, 102–127. [CrossRef] [PubMed]
27. Abdelhafiz, D.; Yang, C.; Ammar, R.; Nabavi, S. Deep convolutional neural networks for mammography: Advances, challenges and applications. *BMC Bioinform.* **2019**, *20*, 281. [CrossRef]
28. Sadik, M.; Hamadeh, I.; Nordblom, P.; Suurkula, M.; Höglund, P.; Ohlsson, M.; Edenbrandt, L. Computer-Assisted Interpretation of Planar Whole-Body Bone Scans. *J. Nucl. Med.* **2008**, *49*, 1958–1965. [CrossRef]
29. Horikoshi, H.; Kikuchi, A.; Onoguchi, M.; Sjöstrand, K.; Edenbrandt, L. Computer-aided diagnosis system for bone scintigrams from Japanese patients: Importance of training database. *Ann. Nucl. Med.* **2012**, *26*, 622–626. [CrossRef] [PubMed]
30. Koizumi, M.; Miyaji, N.; Murata, T.; Motegi, K.; Miwa, K.; Koyama, M.; Terauchi, T.; Wagatsuma, K.; Kawakami, K.; Richter, J. Evaluation of a revised version of computer-assisted diagnosis system, BONENAVI version 2.1.7, for bone scintigraphy in cancer patients. *Ann. Nucl. Med.* **2015**, *29*, 659–665. [CrossRef]
31. Komeda, Y.; Handa, H.; Watanabe, T.; Nomura, T.; Kitahashi, M.; Sakurai, T.; Okamoto, A.; Minami, T.; Kono, M.; Arizumi, T.; et al. Computer-Aided Diagnosis Based on Convolutional Neural Network System for Colorectal Polyp Classification: Preliminary Experience. *Oncology* **2017**, *93*, 30–34. [CrossRef]
32. Shen, D.; Wu, G.; Suk, H.-I. Deep Learning in Medical Image Analysis. *Annu. Rev. Biomed. Eng.* **2017**, *19*, 221–248. [CrossRef]

33. Papandrianos, N.; Papageorgiou, E.; Anagnostis, A.; Feleki, A. A Deep-Learning Approach for Diagnosis of Metastatic Breast Cancer in Bones from Whole-Body Scans. *Appl. Sci.* **2020**, *10*, 997. [CrossRef]
34. Xue, Y.; Chen, S.; Qin, J.; Liu, Y.; Huang, B.; Chen, H. Application of Deep Learning in Automated Analysis of Molecular Images in Cancer: A Survey. *Contrast Media Mol. Imaging* **2017**, *2017*, 1–10. [CrossRef] [PubMed]
35. LeCun, Y.; Bottou, L.; Bengio, Y.; Haffner, P. Gradient-based learning applied to document recognition. *Proc. IEEE* **1998**, *86*, 2278–2324. [CrossRef]
36. LeCun, Y.; Jackel, L.; Bottou, L.; Cortes, C.; Denker, J.; Drucker, H.; Guyon, I.; Muller, U.; Sackinger, E.; Simard, P.; et al. Learning Algorithms for Classification: A Comparison on Handwritten Digit Recognition. 1995. Available online: http://yann.lecun.com/exdb/publis/pdf/lecun-95a.pdf (accessed on 7 July 2021).
37. Qian, N. On the momentum term in gradient descent learning algorithms. *Neural Netw.* **1999**, *12*, 145–151. [CrossRef]
38. Zeiler, M.D.; Fergus, R. Visualizing and Understanding Convolutional Networks BT—Computer Vision–ECCV 2014. In *Proceedings of the European Conference on Computer Vision (ECCV)*; Springer: Berlin/Heidelberg, Germany, 2014; pp. 818–833.
39. Simonyan, K.; Zisserman, A. Very deep convolutional networks for large-scale image recognition. *arXiv* **2014**, arXiv:1409.1556.
40. Guerra, E.; de Lara, J.; Malizia, A.; Díaz, P. Supporting user-oriented analysis for multi-view domain-specific visual languages. *Inf. Softw. Technol.* **2009**, *51*, 769–784. [CrossRef]
41. Szegedy, C.; Liu, W.; Jia, Y.; Sermanet, P.; Reed, S.; Anguelov, D.; Erhan, D.; Vanhoucke, V.; Rabinovich, A. Going Deeper with Convolutions. In Proceedings of the IEEE Conference on Computer Vision and Pattern Recognition (CVPR), Boston, MA, USA, 7–12 June 2015; pp. 1–9.
42. He, K.; Zhang, X.; Ren, S.; Sun, J. Deep residual learning for image recognition. In Proceedings of the 2016 IEEE Conference on Computer Vision and Pattern Recognition, Las Vegas, NV, USA, 27–30 June 2016; pp. 770–778.
43. Huang, G.; Liu, Z.; Van Der Maaten, L.; Weinberger, K.Q. Densely Connected Convolutional Networks. In Proceedings of the 2017 IEEE Conference on Computer Vision and Pattern Recognition (CVPR), Honolulu, HI, USA, 21–26 July 2017; pp. 2261–2269.
44. Arsanjani, R.; Xu, Y.; Dey, D.; Vahistha, V.; Shalev, A.; Nakanishi, R.; Hayes, S.; Fish, M.; Berman, D.; Germano, G.; et al. Improved accuracy of myocardial perfusion SPECT for detection of coronary artery disease by machine learning in a large population. *J. Nucl. Cardiol.* **2013**, *20*, 553–562. [CrossRef] [PubMed]
45. Hu, L.-H.; Betancur, J.; Sharir, T.; Einstein, A.J.; Bokhari, S.; Fish, M.B.; Ruddy, T.D.; A Kaufmann, P.; Sinusas, A.J.; Miller, E.J.; et al. Machine learning predicts per-vessel early coronary revascularization after fast myocardial perfusion SPECT: Results from multicentre REFINE SPECT registry. *Eur. Hear. J. Cardiovasc. Imaging* **2020**, *21*, 549–559. [CrossRef]
46. Lomsky, M.; Gjertsson, P.; Johansson, L.; Richter, J.; Ohlsson, M.; Tout, D.; Van Aswegen, A.; Underwood, S.R.; Edenbrandt, L. Evaluation of a decision support system for interpretation of myocardial perfusion gated SPECT. *Eur. J. Nucl. Med. Mol. Imaging* **2008**, *35*, 1523–1529. [CrossRef]
47. Rahmani, R.; Niazi, P.; Naseri, M.; Neishabouri, M.; Farzanefar, S.; Eftekhari, M.; Derakhshan, F.; Mollazadeh, R.; Meysami, A.; Abbasi, M. Precisión diagnóstica mejorada para la imagen de perfusión miocárdica usando redes neuronales artificiales en diferentes variables de entrada incluyendo datos clínicos y de cuantificación. *Rev. Española Med. Nucl. Imagen Mol.* **2019**, *38*, 275–279. [CrossRef] [PubMed]
48. Arsanjani, R.; Xu, Y.; Dey, D.; Fish, M.; Dorbala, S.; Hayes, S.; Berman, D.; Germano, G.; Slomka, P. Improved Accuracy of Myocardial Perfusion SPECT for the Detection of Coronary Artery Disease Using a Support Vector Machine Algorithm. *J. Nucl. Med.* **2013**, *54*, 549–555. [CrossRef] [PubMed]
49. Güner, L.A.; Karabacak, N.I.; Akdemir, O.U.; Karagoz, P.S.; Kocaman, S.A.; Cengel, A.; Ünlü, M. An open-source framework of neural networks for diagnosis of coronary artery disease from myocardial perfusion SPECT. *J. Nucl. Cardiol.* **2010**, *17*, 405–413. [CrossRef]
50. Betancur, J.; Hu, L.-H.; Commandeur, F.; Sharir, T.; Einstein, A.J.; Fish, M.B.; Ruddy, T.D.; Kaufmann, P.A.; Sinusas, A.J.; Miller, E.J.; et al. Deep Learning Analysis of Upright-Supine High-Efficiency SPECT Myocardial Perfusion Imaging for Prediction of Obstructive Coronary Artery Disease: A Multicenter Study. *J. Nucl. Med.* **2018**, *60*, 664–670. [CrossRef] [PubMed]
51. Betancur, J.; Commandeur, F.; Motlagh, M.; Sharir, T.; Einstein, A.J.; Bokhari, S.; Fish, M.B.; Ruddy, T.D.; Kaufmann, P.; Sinusas, A.J.; et al. Deep Learning for Prediction of Obstructive Disease From Fast Myocardial Perfusion SPECT. *JACC: Cardiovasc. Imaging* **2018**, *11*, 1654–1663. [CrossRef] [PubMed]
52. Spier, N.; Nekolla, S.G.; Rupprecht, C.; Mustafa, M.; Navab, N.; Baust, M. Classification of Polar Maps from Cardiac Perfusion Imaging with Graph-Convolutional Neural Networks. *Sci. Rep.* **2019**, *9*, 1–8. [CrossRef] [PubMed]
53. Berkaya, S.K.; Sivrikoz, I.A.; Gunal, S. Classification models for SPECT myocardial perfusion imaging. *Comput. Biol. Med.* **2020**, *123*, 103893. [CrossRef]
54. Verberne, H.J.; Acampa, W.; Anagnostopoulos, C.D.; Ballinger, J.R.; Bengel, F.; De Bondt, P.; Buechel, R.R.; Cuocolo, A.; Van Eck-Smit, B.L.F.; Flotats, A.; et al. EANM procedural guidelines for radionuclide myocardial perfusion imaging with SPECT and SPECT/CT: 2015 revision. *Eur. J. Nucl. Med. Mol. Imaging* **2015**, *42*, 1929–1940. [CrossRef]
55. Arsanjani, R.; Dey, D.; Khachatryan, T.; Shalev, A.; Hayes, S.W.; Fish, M.; Nakanishi, R.; Germano, G.; Berman, D.S.; Slomka, P. Prediction of revascularization after myocardial perfusion SPECT by machine learning in a large population. *J. Nucl. Cardiol.* **2014**, *22*, 877–884. [CrossRef]
56. Papandrianos, N.; Papageorgiou, E.; Anagnostis, A.; Papageorgiou, K. Bone metastasis classification using whole body images from prostate cancer patients based on convolutional neural networks application. *PLoS ONE* **2020**, *15*, e0237213. [CrossRef]

57. Papandrianos, N.; Papageorgiou, E.I.; Anagnostis, A. Development of Convolutional Neural Networks to identify bone metastasis for prostate cancer patients in bone scintigraphy. *Ann. Nucl. Med.* **2020**, *34*, 824–832. [CrossRef]
58. Papandrianos, N.; Papageorgiou, E.; Anagnostis, A.; Papageorgiou, K. Efficient Bone Metastasis Diagnosis in Bone Scintigraphy Using a Fast Convolutional Neural Network Architecture. *Diagnostics* **2020**, *10*, 532. [CrossRef]
59. Papandrianos, N.; Alexiou, S.; Xouria, X.; Apostolopoulos, D.J. Atypical Bilateral Stress Fractures of the Femoral Shaft Diagnosed by Bone Scintigraphy in a Woman With Osteoporosis. *Clin. Nucl. Med.* **2013**, *38*, 910–912. [CrossRef]
60. O'Shea, K.T.; Nash, R. An Introduction to Convolutional Neural Networks. *arXiv* **2015**, arXiv:1511.08458.
61. Springenberg, J.T.; Dosovitskiy, A.; Brox, T.; Riedmiller, M. Striving for simplicity: The all convolutional net. *arXiv* **2014**, arXiv:1412.6806.
62. Yamashita, R.; Nishio, M.; Do, R.K.G.; Togashi, K. Convolutional neural networks: An overview and application in radiology. *Insights Imaging* **2018**, *9*, 611–629. [CrossRef] [PubMed]
63. Russakovsky, O.; Deng, J.; Su, H.; Krause, J.; Satheesh, S.; Ma, S.; Huang, Z.; Karpathy, A.; Khosla, A.; Bernstein, M.; et al. ImageNet Large Scale Visual Recognition Challenge. *Int. J. Comput. Vis.* **2015**, *115*, 211–252. [CrossRef]
64. Deng, J.; Dong, W.; Socher, R.; Li, L.-J.; Li, K.; Li, F.-F. ImageNet: A large-scale hierarchical image database. In Proceedings of the 2009 IEEE Computer Society Conference on Computer Vision and Pattern Recognition Workshops, Miami, FL, USA, 20–25 June 2009; pp. 248–255.
65. Colaboratory Cloud Environment Supported by Google. Available online: https://colab.research.google.com/ (accessed on 7 July 2021).

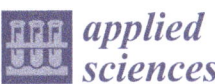

Article

Deep Learning Based Airway Segmentation Using Key Point Prediction

Jinyoung Park [1,†], JaeJoon Hwang [2,3,†], Jihye Ryu [1], Inhye Nam [1], Sol-A Kim [1], Bong-Hae Cho [2,3], Sang-Hun Shin [1,3] and Jae-Yeol Lee [1,3,*]

1. Department of Oral and Maxillofacial Surgery, School of Dentistry, Pusan National University, Yangsan 50612, Korea; forfind@pusan.ac.kr (J.P.); ryujh@umich.edu (J.R.); namih0220@pusan.ac.kr (I.N.); sol3926@pusan.ac.kr (S.-A.K.); ssh8080@pusan.ac.kr (S.-H.S.)
2. Department of Oral and Maxillofacial Radiology, School of Dentistry, Pusan National University, Yangsan 50612, Korea; softdent@pusan.ac.kr (J.H.); bhjo@pusan.ac.kr (B.-H.C.)
3. Dental and Life Science Institute & Dental Research Institute, School of Dentistry, Pusan National University, Yangsan 50612, Korea
* Correspondence: omsljy@pusan.ac.kr; Tel.: +82-55-360-5111
† Jinyoung Park and JaeJoon Hwang have equally contributed to this work and should be considered co-first authors.

Abstract: The purpose of this study was to investigate the accuracy of the airway volume measurement by a Regression Neural Network-based deep-learning model. A set of manually outlined airway data was set to build the algorithm for fully automatic segmentation of a deep learning process. Manual landmarks of the airway were determined by one examiner using a mid-sagittal plane of cone-beam computed tomography (CBCT) images of 315 patients. Clinical dataset-based training with data augmentation was conducted. Based on the annotated landmarks, the airway passage was measured and segmented. The accuracy of our model was confirmed by measuring the following between the examiner and the program: (1) a difference in volume of nasopharynx, oropharynx, and hypopharynx, and (2) the Euclidean distance. For the agreement analysis, 61 samples were extracted and compared. The correlation test showed a range of good to excellent reliability. A difference between volumes were analyzed using regression analysis. The slope of the two measurements was close to 1 and showed a linear regression correlation (r^2 = 0.975, slope = 1.02, $p < 0.001$). These results indicate that fully automatic segmentation of the airway is possible by training via deep learning of artificial intelligence. Additionally, a high correlation between manual data and deep learning data was estimated.

Keywords: airway volume analysis; deep learning; artificial intelligence

1. Introduction

Recently, artificial intelligence has been used in the medical field to predict risk factors through correlation analysis and genomic analyses, phenotype-genotype association studies, and automated medical image analysis [1]. Recent advances in machine learning are contributing to research on identifying, classifying, and quantifying medical image patterns in deep learning. Since the convolutional neural network (CNN) based on artificial neural networks has begun to be used in medical image analysis, research on various diseases is rapidly increasing [2,3]. The use of deep learning in the medical field helps diagnose and treat diseases by extracting and analyzing medical images, and its effectiveness has been proven [4].

However, studies related to deep learning in the areas of oral and maxillofacial surgery are limited [5]. For oral and maxillofacial surgery, radiology is used as an important evaluation criterion in the diagnosis of diseases, treatment plans, and follow-up after treatment. However, the evaluation process is performed manually and the assessment can be different among examiners, or even with the same examiner. This may result in an inefficient and time-consuming procedure [6]. In particular, the evaluation of the airway is difficult to analyze due to its anatomical complexity and the limited difference in gray scale between soft tissue and air [7–9]. Airway analysis is essential for diagnosis and assessment of the treatment progress of obstructive sleep apnea patients and for predicting the tendency of airway changes after orthognathic surgery [10–21].

In most previous studies, the airway was segmented semi-automatically using software systems for volumetric measurements using cone-beam computed tomography (CBCT) images [21–23]. These studies evaluated the reliability and reproducibility of the software systems on the measurement of the airway [7,24–27] and compared the accuracy between the various software systems [9,24,25,27]. However, in all cases, the software systems require manual processing by experts.

In this study, a regression neural network-based deep-learning model is proposed, which will enable fully automatic segmentation of airways using CBCT. The differences between the manually measured data and data measured by deep learning will be analyzed. Using a manually positioned data set, training and deep learning will be performed to determine the possibility of a fully automatic segmentation of the airway and to introduce a method and its proposed future use.

2. Materials and Methods

2.1. Sample Collection and Information

Images from 315 patients who underwent CBCT for orthognathic surgery were collected retrospectively from 2017 to 2019. The CBCT data were acquired using PaX-i3D (Vatech Co., Hwaseong-si, Korea) at 105–114 KVP, 5.6–6.5 mA with 160 mm × 160 mm field of view, and 0.3 mm in voxel size. The scanning conditions were automatically determined by the machine according to the patients' age and gender. The CBCT images were converted to DICOM 3.0 and stored on a Windows-10-based graphic workstation (Intel Core i7-4770, 32 GB). The patients were all placed in a natural head position. All image processing was performed using MATLAB 2020a (MathWorks, Natick, MA, USA) programming language.

2.2. Coordinate Determination in the Mid-Sagittal Plane

Five coordinates for each original image were obtained manually in the midsagittal plane of the CBCT images (Figure 1). The definitions of the points and planes for the airway division are presented in Table 1, referring to Lee et al. [28]. These five coordinates were predicted by a 2D convolutional neural network for airway segmentation in the sagittal direction.

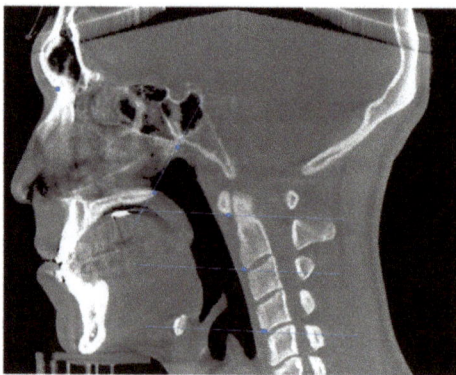

Figure 1. Coordinate and plane determination in the midsagittal plane of the cone-beam computed tomography (CBCT) image.

Table 1. Definition of reference points and planes for airway division. (Abbreviations: PNS, posterior nasal spine; VP, posterior point of vomer; CV1, 1st cervical vertebra; CV2, 2nd cervical vertebra; CV4, 4th cervical vertebra).

Definition	Explanation
Reference Points	
PNS	Most posterior point of palate
VP	Most posterior point of vomer
CV1	Most anterior inferior point of anterior arch of atlas
CV2	Most anterior inferior point of anterior arch of second vertebra
CV4	Most anterior inferior point of anterior arch of fourth vertebra
Reference planes	
PNS-Vp plane	The plane was perpendicular to the midsagittal plane passing through the PNS and the Vp.
CV1 plane	The plane was parallel to the natural head position plane passing through CV1.
CV2 plane	The plane was parallel to the natural head position plane passing through CV2.
CV3 plane	The plane was parallel to the natural head position plane passing through CV3.
CV4 plane	The plane was parallel to the natural head position plane passing through CV4.
Volume	
Nasopharynx	From PNS-VP plane to CV1 plane
Oropharynx	From CV1 plane to CV2 plane
Hypopharynx	From CV2 plane to CV4 plane

2.3. Airway Segmentation

First, the image was binarized, then it was filled through a 3D close operation, and hole filling, and then, the binarized image was subtracted from the filled image to obtain an airway image. After erasing the image outside, the area that references five points, and the 1/4 and 3/4 of the inferior border are connected. Only the largest object is left to obtain the airway image (Figure 2).

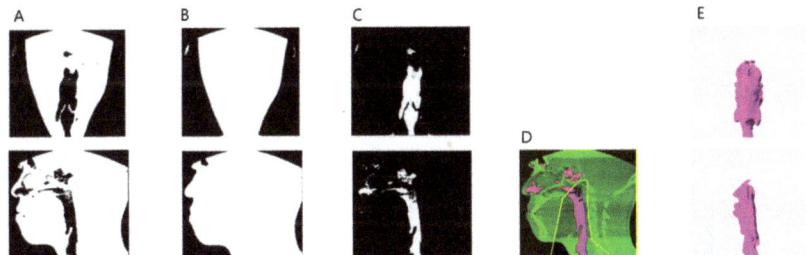

Figure 2. Airway segmentation process. (**A**) Binarization image. (**B**) Hole filled image after close operation. (**C**) Difference image between (**A**,**B**). (**D**) An image that erases the area outside the area where 5 reference points, and 1/4 and 3/4 of the inferior border are connected. (**E**) Segmented airway.

2.4. Training via Regression Neural Network and Metrics for Accuracy Comparison

The 315 midsagittal images obtained from the patient's cone-beam computed tomography (CBCT) data were split into training and test sets at a ratio of 4:1. During clinical data set-based training, validation was not performed because the sample size was too small for validation. Instead, a five-fold cross-validation was applied. First, the image size was set to 200 × 200 pixels, and 16 convolution layers were packed for feature extraction. To generate the regression model, the regression layer was connected to a fully connected layer. Mean-squared-error was used as a loss function. Data augmentation was then conducted, including rotation from −6° to +6°, uniform (isotropic) scaling from 0.5° to 1°, Poisson noise addition, and contrast and brightness adjustment. An NVIDIA Titan RTX GPU with CUDA (version 10.1) acceleration was used for network training. The models were trained for 243 epochs using an Adam optimizer with an initial learning rate of 1e-4 and a mini-batch size of 8.

The prediction accuracy of the model was calculated using (a) the volume difference between the predicted and manually determined nasopharynx, oropharynx, and hypopharynx, and (b) the Euclidean distance between where the predicted and manually determined points are real data.

3. Results

3.1. Measurements of the Differences between Manual Analysis and Deep Learning Analysis

The five coordinates manually pointed and predicted by the deep learning model are shown in Figure 3. The Euclidean distance between the predicted and manually determined points was largest at CV4 (4.156 ± 2.379 mm) and smallest at CV1 (2.571 ± 2.028 mm). Other Euclidean distances were estimated as 2.817 ± 1.806 mm at PNS, 2.837 ± 1.924 mm at Vp, and 2.896 ± 2.205 mm at CV2. When the volume was compared for each part, the hypopharynx showed the largest difference difference (50 ± 57.891 mm^3), and the oropharynx was assessed as having the smallest difference (37.987 ± 43.289 mm^3). The difference in the nasopharyngeal area was 48.620 ± 49.468 mm^3. The difference in total volume was measured as 137.256 ± 146.517 mm^3. All measurements of the differences are shown in Table 2. Volume differences among parts of the airway are shown in Figure 4.

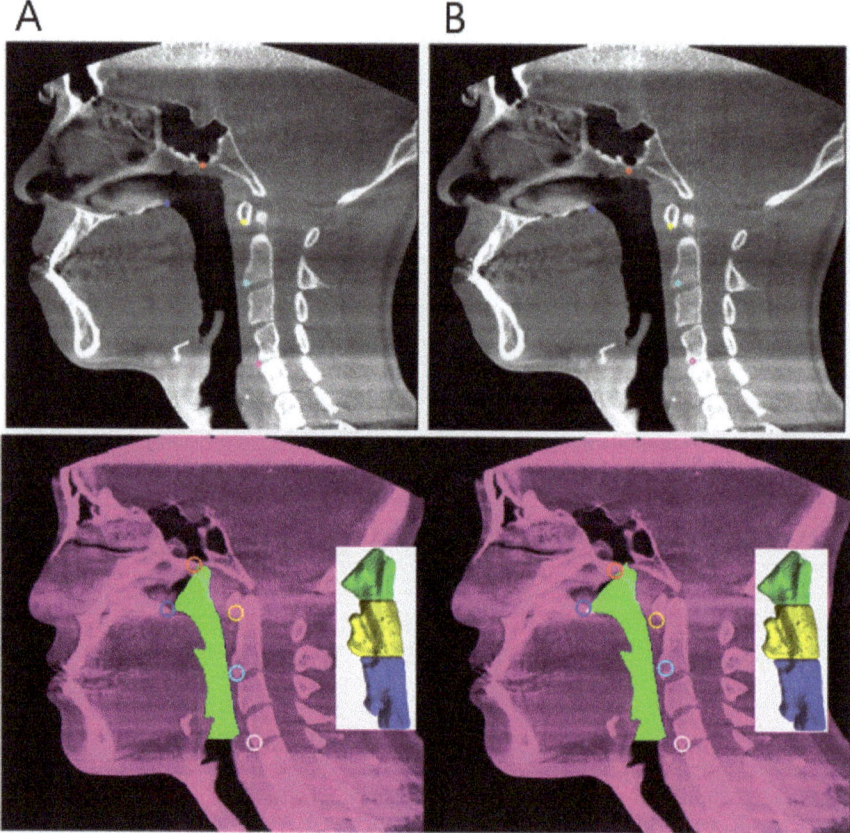

Figure 3. (**A**) Example of manually pointed data and its volume segmentation. (**B**) Example of deep learning pointed data and its volume segmentation.

Table 2. Measurements of the differences between manual analysis and deep learning analysis (N = 61).

	Average	SD
Volume (mm^3)		
Nasopharynx	48.620	49.468
Oropharynx	37.987	43.289
Hypopharynx	50.010	57.891
Total volume	85.256	86.504
Distances between M and DL (mm)		
PNS	2.817	1.806
VP	2.837	1.924
CV1	2.571	2.028
CV2	2.896	2.205
CV4	4.156	2.379

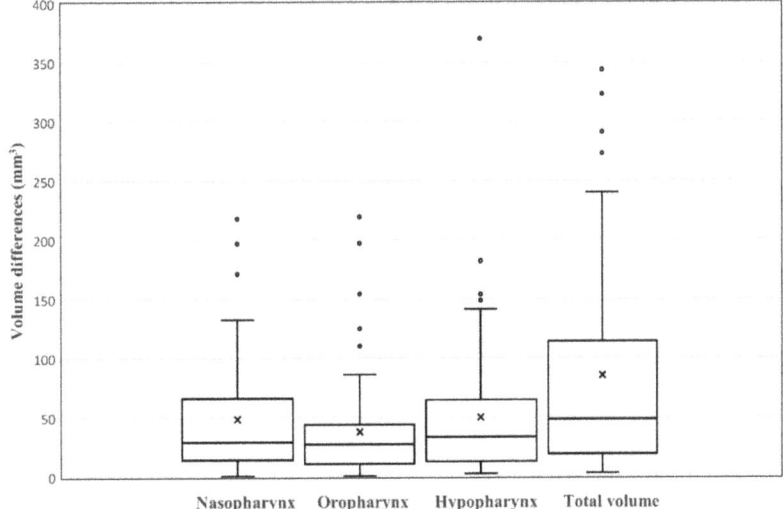

Figure 4. Boxplots of the differences between manual analysis and deep learning analysis (N = 61). In the boxplots, 'x' within the box marks the mean of volume differences.

3.2. Agreement Analysis

Using agreement analysis, 61 samples were extracted and the manually measured value and deep learning network predicted value were compared for both volumes and coordinates. The total volume was the most correlated intra-class correlation coefficient (ICC) value in the oropharynx (0.986), followed by the hypopharynx (0.964), and the nasopharynx (0.912). The intra-class correlation coefficient (ICC) value for the coordinate CV2(x) was the most correlated (0.963) and the least correlated at CV4(y) (0.868). All ICC values are presented in Table 3.

Table 3. Agreement analysis of the volume and point via intra-class correlation coefficient (ICC) (Two-way random effects, absolute agreement, single rater/measurement) (N = 61).

Variables	ICC	95% CI	
		Lower Limit	Upper Limit
Volume			
Nasopharynx	0.912	0.858	0.946
Oropharynx	0.984	0.973	0.99
Hypopharynx	0.964	0.941	0.978
Total volume	0.986	0.977	0.992
Coordinate			
PNS(x)	0.908	0.852	0.944
PNS(y)	0.952	0.921	0.971
Vp(x)	0.908	0.842	0.946
Vp(y)	0.939	0.89	0.965
CV1(x)	0.929	0.885	0.957
CV1(y)	0.956	0.928	0.974
CV2(x)	0.963	0.939	0.978
CV2(y)	0.924	0.877	0.954
CV4(x)	0.953	0.924	0.972
CV4(y)	0.868	0.79	0.919

3.3. Linear Regression Scatter Plots and Bland-Altman Plot for the Total Volume Data Set

The total volume measured by deep learning was compared with the volume manually measured using regression analysis (Figure 5). The slopes of the two measurements were close to 1 and showed a linear regression correlation as $r^2 = 0.975$, slope = 1.02, and $p < 0.001$. Bland-Altman plots and analyses were used to compare the total volume of the two methods, and the results are presented in Figure 6. The Bland-Altman plot comparing the level of agreement between manual and deep learning indicates an upper limit of agreement (0.261 cm^3) and a lower limit of agreement (−0.207 cm^3). The range of the 95% confidence interval was 0.468 cm^3.

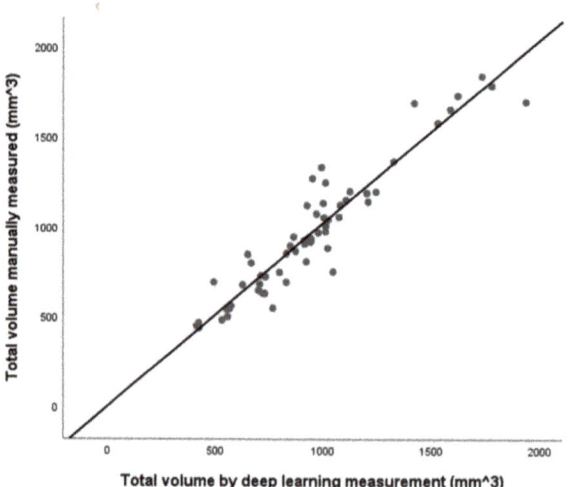

Figure 5. Scatter plot of total volume measured between the manual of deep learning ($r^2 = 0.975$, slope = 1.02, $p < 0.001$). The line indicates a linear regression graph. There is a strong correlation between the two methods (N = 61).

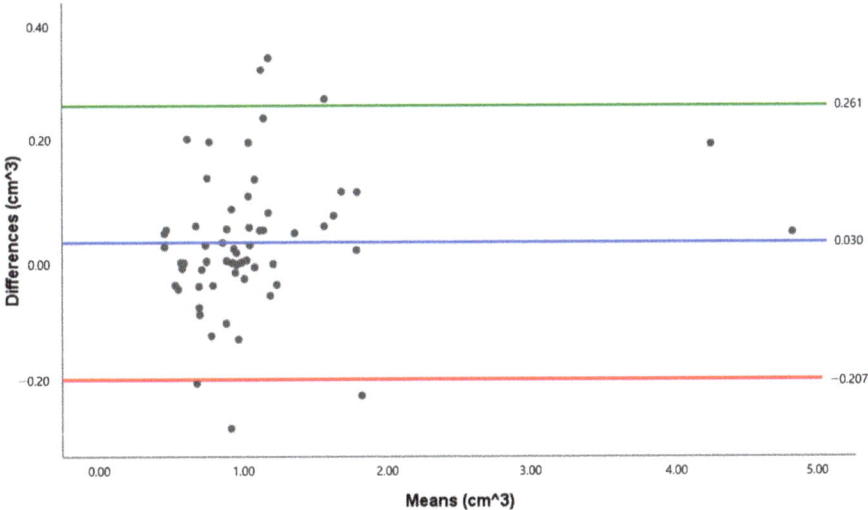

Figure 6. Bland-Altman plot of the total volume data set. The green line indicates the upper limit of agreement, while the red line indicates the lower limit of agreement (N = 61).

4. Discussion

In the medical field, many studies have used artificial intelligence via deep learning in radiology [29,30]. There are studies on fully automated airway segmentation of lungs with volumetric computed tomographic images using a convolutional neural network (CNN) [31] and on automatic segmentation and 3D reconstruction of inferior turbinate and maxillary sinus from otorhinolaryngology [32]. Due to the complex anatomical structure of the airway, there are difficulties in researching the airway using manual measurements, which is a time-consuming process, and entails inter-examiner error, intra-examiner error, and a lack of certainty because of the small differences on a gray scale [23]. For these reasons, automated measurement and analysis are necessary, but the fully auto-segmentation of the airway is challenging and a study of airway segmentation using deep learning in the area of oral and maxillofacial surgery has not previously been reported.

Therefore, in this study, we performed a fully automated segmentation of the airway using artificial intelligence for enabling faster and more practical measurement and analysis in clinical practice. The correlation between the coordinates and volumes measured manually and by the deep learning network were evaluated and compared. The distance between the coordinates of each of the five airway reference points was measured between 2.5 mm and 4.1 mm, and the difference between the measured volumes was 48.620 mm^3 in the nasopharynx, 37.987 mm^3 in the oropharynx, and 50.010 mm^3 in the hypopharynx. The difference in total volume was observed to be 85.256 mm^3. Therefore, it is considered that the correlation between each coordinate and volume showed good to excellent reliability.

In this study, the threshold is defined by the Otsu method [33], the binarized image is extracted, and deep learning performs fully automatic division of the airway and divides it into the nasopharynx, oropharynx, and hypopharynx parts through the reference plane.

The difference between the total volumes in this study was evaluated as an acceptable value at 0.46 cm^3 when compared to the Torres et al. [25] study, which gave the difference between the water volume of an actual prototype and the volume on the CT software as 0.2 cm^3 to 1.0 cm^3. The difference in the volume of the oropharynx was measured as the smallest, which showed the same results as El et al. [34]. According to Alsufyani et al. [23], since the oropharynx airway is a completely empty space like a tube, it is straightforward to measure the volume. The more complex and narrow shape of the airway's soft tissue is due to anatomical complexity, such as epiglottis. This has the highest error in volumetric measurements [35]. Therefore, it can be considered that a simpler anatomical structure will result in a smaller difference between the measurement methods.

When comparing the distance of each point, the result of this study is not clinically applicable. A clinically acceptable difference between the landmarks is approximately 2 mm, according to Lee et al. [36]. There are several reasons for a possible error, which include the limitation in the number of training data sets and the necessity for more precise data preparation, such as setting more reference points on each slice segmentation. In setting the reference points for precise training, the reference points were selected on the bony parts to reduce the error due to the variety of soft tissue shapes. This allows clear determination of the anatomical point aided by the large difference on a gray scale, and a simpler comparison of the relationship before and after surgery. Hence, this study applied the reference points of the Lee et al. study [28]. Nevertheless, in the present study, the distance of CV4 had a larger error, which may be due to the shape of the spine CV4 appearing in various ways in the sagittal plane compared to CV1 or CV2. It is necessary to set an additional reference point to define the hypopharynx that appears to be constant in the midsagittal plane.

The limitation of most airway segmentation research is possibly due to an inconsistent patient head position [23,27,37]. Since patients underwent CBCT in the natural head position in this study, errors may occur. It has been reported that the shape of the airway can vary greatly depending on the angle of the head [38]. However, as concluded in most research, it is not a significant error when comparing the volume of the airway rather than evaluating the volume itself [25]. When performing CBCT, the patient's head position is consistently adjusted to a natural head position by the examiner through the head strap, chin support, and guide light. In addition, the natural head position has been proven to be reproducible [39], and, hence, there should be no major error when comparing. Due to breathing and tongue position, errors may occur in volumetric measurements [35,37]. Therefore, for each variable, controlled and consistent scanning is required. This study divided the airway volume using 5 points in the 2D mid-sagittal image. The accuracy of these points affects the accuracy of airway segmentation. Therefore, bigger data is needed for clinical application of our algorithm to raise accuracy of coordinate determination.

In the agreement analysis, according to Koo et al. [40], "Based on the 95% confident interval of the ICC estimate, values less than 0.5, between 0.5 and 0.75, between 0.75 and 0.90, and greater than 0.90 are indicative of poor, moderate, good, and excellent reliability, respectively." In the present study, oropharynx, hypopharynx, total volume, PNS(y), CV1(y), CV2(x), and CV4(x) indicated excellent reliability, and all other variables indicated good reliability based on the Koo et al. report [40].

These results indicate that fully automatic segmentation of the airway is possible through training via deep learning of artificial intelligence. In addition, high correlation between manual data and deep learning data was estimated. To improve the accuracy, validity, and reliability of auto-segmentation, further data collection and optimum training with big data will be required for future clinical application. Furthermore, to raise the robustness of our algorithm, bigger data is needed for accurate coordinate determination. Transfer learning with other datasets, such as facial coordinates, can also be useful. We plan to develop more robust algorithms with bigger data.

5. Conclusions

In this study, using a manually positioned data set, fully automatic segmentation of the airway was possible with artificial intelligence by training a deep learning algorithm and a high correlation between manual data and deep learning data was estimated.

As the first study to utilize artificial intelligence to reach full auto-segmentation of the airway, this paper is meaningful in showing the possibility of a more accurate and quicker way of producing airway segmentation. For a future clinical application, the more robust algorithms with bigger and multiplex datasets are required.

Author Contributions: J.P. and J.H. carried out the analysis of data and prepared the manuscript. J.R. and I.N. helped in the collection and analysis of the data. S.-AK. helped the visualization and analysis of the data in a revised manuscript. B.-H.C. and S.-H.S. conceived of the study, participated in its design and coordination, and helped to draft the manuscript. J.-Y.L. designed the study and drafted the manuscript. All authors have read and agreed to the published version of the manuscript.

Funding: This research was supported by a grant of the Korea Health Technology R&D Project through the Korea Health Industry Development Institute (KHIDI), funded by the Ministry of Health & Welfare, Republic of Korea (grant number: HI19C0824).

Institutional Review Board Statement: The study was conducted according to the guidelines of the Declaration of Helsinki, and approved by the Institutional Review Board of Pusan National Dental Hospital (PNUDH-2021-008).

Informed Consent Statement: Patient consent was waived because of the retrospective nature of the study and the analysis used anonymous clinical data.

Data Availability Statement: The data presented in this study are openly available in Github at: https://github.com/JaeJoonHwang/airway_segmentation_using_key_point_prediction, accessed on 13 April 2021.

Conflicts of Interest: The authors declare no conflict of interest.

References

1. Yu, K.H.; Beam, A.L.; Kohane, I.S. Artificial intelligence in healthcare. *Nat. Biomed. Eng.* **2018**, *2*, 719–731. [CrossRef] [PubMed]
2. LeCun, Y.; Bengio, Y.; Hinton, G. Deep learning. *Nature* **2015**, *521*, 436–444. [CrossRef] [PubMed]
3. Anwar, S.M.; Majid, M.; Qayyum, A.; Awais, M.; Alnowami, M.; Khan, M.K. Medical Image Analysis using Convolutional Neural Networks: A Review. *J. Med. Syst.* **2018**, *42*, 226. [CrossRef] [PubMed]
4. El Naqa, I.; Haider, M.A.; Giger, M.L.; Ten Haken, R.K. Artificial Intelligence: Reshaping the practice of radiological sciences in the 21st century. *Br. J. Radiol.* **2020**, *93*, 20190855. [CrossRef] [PubMed]
5. Fourcade, A.; Khonsari, R.H. Deep learning in medical image analysis: A third eye for doctors. *J. Stomatol. Oral Maxillofac. Surg.* **2019**, *120*, 279–288. [CrossRef] [PubMed]
6. Cho, Y.S.; Cho, K.; Park, C.J.; Chung, M.J.; Kim, J.H.; Kim, K.; Kim, Y.K.; Kim, H.J.; Ko, J.W.; Cho, B.H.; et al. Automated measurement of hydrops ratio from MRI in patients with Meniere's disease using CNN-based segmentation. *Sci. Rep.* **2020**, *10*. [CrossRef] [PubMed]
7. De Water, V.R.; Saridin, J.K.; Bouw, F.; Murawska, M.M.; Koudstaal, M.J. Measuring Upper Airway Volume: Accuracy and Reliability of Dolphin 3D Software Compared to Manual Segmentation in Craniosynostosis Patients. *J. Stomatol. Oral Maxillofac. Surg.* **2014**, *72*, 139–144. [CrossRef] [PubMed]
8. Alsufyani, N.A.; Hess, A.; Noga, M.; Ray, N.; Al-Saleh, M.A.Q.; Lagravere, M.O.; Major, P.W. New algorithm for semiautomatic segmentation of nasal cavity and pharyngeal airway in comparison with manual segmentation using cone-beam computed tomography. *Am. J. Orthod. Dentofac.* **2016**, *150*, 703–712. [CrossRef]
9. Weissheimer, A.; de Menezes, L.M.; Sameshima, G.T.; Enciso, R.; Pham, J.; Grauer, D. Imaging software accuracy for 3-dimensional analysis of the upper airway. *Am. J. Orthod. Dentofac.* **2012**, *142*, 801–813. [CrossRef]
10. Ruckschloss, T.; Ristow, O.; Berger, M.; Engel, M.; Freudlsperger, C.; Hoffmann, J.; Seeberger, R. Relations between mandible-only advancement surgery, the extent of the posterior airway space, and the position of the hyoid bone in Class II patients: A three-dimensional analysis. *Br. J. Oral Maxillofac. Surg.* **2019**, *57*, 1032–1038. [CrossRef]
11. Ruckschloss, T.; Ristow, O.; Jung, A.; Roser, C.; Pilz, M.; Engel, M.; Hoffmann, J.; Seeberger, R. The relationship between bimaxillary orthognathic surgery and the extent of posterior airway space in class II and III patients—A retrospective three-dimensional cohort analysis. *J. Oral Maxillofac. Pathol.* **2021**, *33*, 30–38. [CrossRef]
12. Kamano, E.; Terajima, M.; Kitahara, T.; Takahashi, I. Three-dimensional analysis of changes in pharyngeal airway space after mandibular setback surgery. *Orthod. Waves* **2017**, *76*, 1–8. [CrossRef]
13. Jang, S.I.; Ahn, J.; Paeng, J.Y.; Hong, J. Three-dimensional analysis of changes in airway space after bimaxillary orthognathic surgery with maxillomandibular setback and their association with obstructive sleep apnea. *Maxillofac. Plast. Reconstr. Surg.* **2018**, *40*, 33. [CrossRef]
14. Kim, S.C.; Min, K.; Jeong, W.S.; Kwon, S.M.; Koh, K.S.; Choi, J.W. Three-Dimensional Analysis of Airway Change After LeFort III Midface Advancement with Distraction. *Ann. Plast. Surg.* **2018**, *80*, 359–363. [CrossRef]
15. Niu, X.W.; Di Carlo, G.; Cornelis, M.A.; Cattaneo, P.M. Three-dimensional analyses of short- and long-term effects of rapid maxillary expansion on nasal cavity and upper airway: A systematic review and meta-analysis. *Orthod. Craniofac. Res.* **2020**, *23*, 250–276. [CrossRef]

16. Yamashita, A.L.; Iwaki, L.; Leite, P.C.C.; Navarro, R.D.; Ramos, A.L.; Previdelli, I.T.S.; Ribeiro, M.H.D.; Iwaki, L.C.V. Three-dimensional analysis of the pharyngeal airway space and hyoid bone position after orthognathic surgery. *J. Craniomaxillofac. Surg.* **2017**, *45*, 1408–1414. [CrossRef]
17. Wen, X.; Wang, X.Y.; Qin, S.Q.; Franchi, L.; Gu, Y. Three-dimensional analysis of upper airway morphology in skeletal Class III patients with and without mandibular asymmetry. *Angle Orthod.* **2017**, *87*, 526–533. [CrossRef]
18. Louro, R.S.; Calasans-Maia, J.A.; Mattos, C.T.; Masterson, D.; Calasans-Maia, M.D.; Maia, L.C. Three-dimensional changes to the upper airway after maxillomandibular advancement with counterclockwise rotation: A systematic review and meta-analysis. *Int. J. Oral Maxillofac. Surg.* **2018**, *47*, 622–629. [CrossRef]
19. Tan, S.K.; Tang, A.T.H.; Leung, W.K.; Zwahlen, R.A. Three-Dimensional Pharyngeal Airway Changes After 2-Jaw Orthognathic Surgery with Segmentation in Dento-Skeletal Class III Patients. *J. Craniofac. Surg.* **2019**, *30*, 1533–1538. [CrossRef]
20. Christovam, I.O.; Lisboa, C.O.; Ferreira, D.M.T.P.; Cury-Saramago, A.A.; Mattos, C.T. Upper airway dimensions in patients undergoing orthognathic surgery: A systematic review and meta-analysis. *Int. J. Oral Maxillofac. Surg.* **2016**, *45*, 460–471. [CrossRef]
21. Bianchi, A.; Betti, E.; Tarsitano, A.; Morselli-Labate, A.M.; Lancellotti, L.; Marchetti, C. Volumetric three-dimensional computed tomographic evaluation of the upper airway in patients with obstructive sleep apnoea syndrome treated by maxillomandibular advancement. *Br. J. Oral Maxillofac. Surg.* **2014**, *52*, 831–837. [CrossRef] [PubMed]
22. Stratemann, S.; Huang, J.C.; Maki, K.; Hatcher, D.; Miller, A.J. Three-dimensional analysis of the airway with cone-beam computed tomography. *Am. J. Orthod. Dentofac.* **2011**, *140*, 607–615. [CrossRef] [PubMed]
23. Alsufyani, N.A.; Flores-Mir, C.; Major, P.W. Three-dimensional segmentation of the upper airway using cone beam CT: A systematic review. *Dentomaxillofac. Radiol.* **2012**, *41*, 276–284. [CrossRef] [PubMed]
24. Chen, H.; van Eijnatten, M.; Wolff, J.; de Lange, J.; van der Stelt, P.F.; Lobbezoo, F.; Aarab, G. Reliability and accuracy of three imaging software packages used for 3D analysis of the upper airway on cone beam computed tomography images. *Dentomaxillofac. Radiol.* **2017**, *46*. [CrossRef]
25. Torres, H.M.; Evangelista, K.; Torres, E.M.; Estrela, C.; Leite, A.F.; Valladares-Neto, J.; Silva, M.A.G. Reliability and validity of two software systems used to measure the pharyngeal airway space in three-dimensional analysis. *Int. J. Oral Maxillofac. Surg.* **2020**, *49*, 602–613. [CrossRef]
26. Burkhard, J.P.M.; Dietrich, A.D.; Jacobsen, C.; Roos, M.; Lubbers, H.T.; Obwegeser, J.A. Cephalometric and three-dimensional assessment of the posterior airway space and imaging software reliability analysis before and after orthognathic surgery. *J. Craniomaxillofac. Surg.* **2014**, *42*, 1428–1436. [CrossRef]
27. Zimmerman, J.N.; Lee, J.; Pliska, B.T. Reliability of upper pharyngeal airway assessment using dental CBCT: A systematic review. *Eur. J. Orthodont.* **2017**, *39*, 489–496. [CrossRef]
28. Lee, J.Y.; Kim, Y.I.; Hwang, D.S.; Park, S.B. Effect of Maxillary Setback Movement on Upper Airway in Patients with Class III Skeletal Deformities: Cone Beam Computed Tomographic Evaluation. *J. Craniofac. Surg.* **2013**, *24*, 387–391. [CrossRef]
29. Chan, H.P.; Samala, R.K.; Hadjiiski, L.M.; Zhou, C. Deep Learning in Medical Image Analysis. *Adv. Exp. Med. Biol.* **2020**, *1213*, 3–21. [CrossRef]
30. Shen, D.; Wu, G.; Suk, H.I. Deep Learning in Medical Image Analysis. *Annu. Rev. Biomed. Eng.* **2017**, *19*, 221–248. [CrossRef]
31. Yun, J.; Park, J.; Yu, D.; Yi, J.; Lee, M.; Park, H.J.; Lee, J.G.; Seo, J.B.; Kim, N. Improvement of fully automated airway segmentation on volumetric computed tomographic images using a 2.5 dimensional convolutional neural net. *Med. Image Anal.* **2019**, *51*, 13–20. [CrossRef]
32. Kuo, C.F.J.; Leu, Y.S.; Hu, D.J.; Huang, C.C.; Siao, J.J.; Leon, K.B.P. Application of intelligent automatic segmentation and 3D reconstruction of inferior turbinate and maxillary sinus from computed tomography and analyze the relationship between volume and nasal lesion. *Biomed. Signal Process Control* **2020**, *57*, 19. [CrossRef]
33. Otsu, N. Threshold Selection Method from Gray-Level Histograms. *IEEE Trans. Syst. Man Cybern.* **1979**, *9*, 62–66. [CrossRef]
34. El, H.; Palomo, J.M.; Halazonetis, D.J. Measuring the airway in 3 dimensions: A reliability and accuracy study. *Am. J. Orthod. Dentofac.* **2010**, *137*, S50.e1–S50.e9. [CrossRef]
35. Sutthiprapaporn, P.; Tanimoto, K.; Ohtsuka, M.; Nagasaki, T.; Iida, Y.; Katsumata, A. Positional changes of oropharyngeal structures due to gravity in the upright and supine positions. *Dentomaxillofac. Radiol.* **2008**, *37*, 130–135. [CrossRef]
36. Lee, J.H.; Yu, H.J.; Kim, M.J.; Kim, J.W.; Choi, J. Automated cephalometric landmark detection with confidence regions using Bayesian convolutional neural networks. *BMC Oral Health* **2020**, *20*, 270. [CrossRef]
37. Guijarro-Martinez, R.; Swennen, G.R.J. Cone-beam computerized tomography imaging and analysis of the upper airway: A systematic review of the literature. *Int. J. Oral Maxillofac. Surg.* **2011**, *40*, 1227–1237. [CrossRef]
38. Muto, T.; Takeda, S.; Kanazawa, M.; Yamazaki, A.; Fujiwara, Y.; Mizoguchi, I. The effect of head posture on the pharyngeal airway space (PAS). *Int. J. Oral Maxillofac. Surg.* **2002**, *31*, 579–583. [CrossRef]
39. Weber, D.W.; Fallis, D.W.; Packer, M.D. Three-dimensional reproducibility of natural head position. *Am. J. Orthod. Dentofac. Orthop.* **2013**, *143*, 738–744. [CrossRef]
40. Koo, T.K.; Li, M.Y. A Guideline of Selecting and Reporting Intraclass Correlation Coefficients for Reliability Research. *J. Chiropr. Med.* **2016**, *15*, 155–163. [CrossRef]

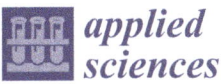

Article

Characterization of Optical Coherence Tomography Images for Colon Lesion Differentiation under Deep Learning

Cristina L. Saratxaga [1,2,*], Jorge Bote [3], Juan F. Ortega-Morán [3], Artzai Picón [1], Elena Terradillos [1], Nagore Arbide del Río [4], Nagore Andraka [5], Estibaliz Garrote [1,6] and Olga M. Conde [2,7,8]

1. TECNALIA, Basque Research and Technology Alliance (BRTA), Parque Científico y Tecnológico de Bizkaia, C/Geldo. Edificio 700, 48160 Derio, Spain; artzai.picon@tecnalia.com (A.P.); elena.terradillos@tecnalia.com (E.T.); estibaliz.garrote@tecnalia.com (E.G.)
2. Photonics Engineering Group, University of Cantabria, 39005 Santander, Spain; olga.conde@unican.es
3. Jesús Usón Minimally Invasive Surgery Centre, Ctra. N-521, km 41.8, 10071 Cáceres, Spain; jbote@ccmijesususon.com (J.B.); jfortega@ccmijesususon.com (J.F.O.-M.)
4. Anatomic Pathology Service, Basurto University Hospital, 48013 Bilbao, Spain; nagore.arbidedelrio@osakidetza.eus
5. Basque Foundation for Health Innovation and Research, BEC Tower, Azkue Kalea 1, 48902 Barakaldo, Spain; gestionIDi.biobancovasco@bioef.org
6. Department of Cell Biology and Histology, Faculty of Medicine and Dentistry, University of the Basque Country, 48940 Leioa, Spain
7. Valdecilla Biomedical Research Institute (IDIVAL), 39011 Santander, Spain
8. CIBER-BBN, Biomedical Research Networking Center—Bioengineering, Biomaterials, and Nanomedicine, Avda. Monforte de Lemos, 3–5, Pabellón 11, Planta 0, 28029 Madrid, Spain
* Correspondence: Cristina.lopez@tecnalia.com; Tel.: +34-946-430-850

Featured Application: Automatic diagnosis of colon polyps on optical coherence tomography (OCT) images for the development of computer-aided diagnosis (CADx) applications.

Abstract: (1) Background: Clinicians demand new tools for early diagnosis and improved detection of colon lesions that are vital for patient prognosis. Optical coherence tomography (OCT) allows microscopical inspection of tissue and might serve as an optical biopsy method that could lead to in-situ diagnosis and treatment decisions; (2) Methods: A database of murine (rat) healthy, hyperplastic and neoplastic colonic samples with more than 94,000 images was acquired. A methodology that includes a data augmentation processing strategy and a deep learning model for automatic classification (benign vs. malignant) of OCT images is presented and validated over this dataset. Comparative evaluation is performed both over individual B-scan images and C-scan volumes; (3) Results: A model was trained and evaluated with the proposed methodology using six different data splits to present statistically significant results. Considering this, 0.9695 (±0.0141) sensitivity and 0.8094 (±0.1524) specificity were obtained when diagnosis was performed over B-scan images. On the other hand, 0.9821 (±0.0197) sensitivity and 0.7865 (±0.205) specificity were achieved when diagnosis was made considering all the images in the whole C-scan volume; (4) Conclusions: The proposed methodology based on deep learning showed great potential for the automatic characterization of colon polyps and future development of the optical biopsy paradigm.

Keywords: colon cancer; colon polyps; OCT; deep learning; optical biopsy; animal rat models; CADx

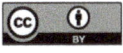

1. Introduction

Colon cancer is the second most common cause of cancer death in Europe both for women and men, and the third most common cancer worldwide [1]. About 1.8 million new cases of colorectal cancer were recorded globally in 2018 [2], being the third most common cancer in men and second in women. The five-year survival rate is 90 percent for colorectal cancers diagnosed at an early stage, but unfortunately only 4 out of 10 cases are found this early [3].

Clinicians demand new non-invasive technologies for early diagnosis of colon polyps, especially to distinguish between benign and malignant or potentially malignant lesions that must be resected immediately. New methods should also proportionate information for safety margin resection and remaining tissue inspection after resection to decrease the possibility of tumor recurrence and improve patient prognosis. The current gold-standard imaging technique during patient examination is colonoscopy with narrow band red-flag technology for improved lesion visualization. During the procedure, lesions can be classified with Paris (morphology) [4] and Nice (vessel and surface) [5] classification patterns based on the physician experience. As this superficial information is not enough, the final diagnosis of the lesion is determined by the histopathological analysis after biopsy, meaning that all the suspicious polyps are resected. Bleeding related problems usually occur after biopsies are performed, with the risks that this entails for the patient. In fact, most problems occur when the biopsy is performed on a blood vessel and the incidence is higher when it is performed on patients with an abnormal blood coagulation function [6]. In relation to the latter, the rate of perforation associated to colonoscopies with polypectomy is 0.8/1000 (95% confidence interval (CI) 0.6–1.0) and the rate of bleeding related to polypectomies is 9.8/1000 (95% confidence interval (CI) 7.7–12.1) [7]. However, it is demonstrated that hyperplastic polyps are of a benign nature and can be left untouched, avoiding the underlying bleeding risk of resection, saving diagnosis time, costs, and patient trauma during that period [8]. On the other side, pre-malignant lesions and adenomatous polyps cannot be distinguished from neoplastic lesions as adenocarcinoma with the current diagnosis methods. In this sense, new imaging techniques and interpretation methods could allow real-time diagnosis and would facilitate better in-situ treatment of lesions, improving patient prognosis, especially if the diagnosis is made at early stages of the disease.

In recent years, different advanced imaging technologies that allow sub-surface microscopical inspection of tissue in an "optical-biopsy" manner have been under study for colonic polyps [9], such as: reflectance confocal microscopy (RCM) [10], multi-photon microscopy (MPM) [11], and optical coherence tomography (OCT) [12], among others. Of the mentioned techniques, a device called Cellvizio based on confocal laser endomicroscopy (CLE) is the only one commercially available. Using confocal mini-probes inserted in the working channel of flexible endoscopes, the system is used for studying the cellular and vascular microarchitecture of tissue. Colorectal lesions diagnosis [13–15] is one of the targeted applications and the corresponding probe reports a field-of-view (FOV) of 240 μm, 1 μm resolution and 55 to 65 μm confocal depth, with 20 maximum uses. The inconvenience of this system is that the successful usage by clinicians depends on specific training on image interpretation. Moreover, the main limitation is that this technology requires the use of an exogenous fluorophore which results in a more invasive procedure for the patient. In the case of MPM [16,17], which relies on the absorption of an external or endogen (as collagen) tissue fluorophore, high resolution images at sub-cellular level can also be obtained to study structural information, including also functional information. The mentioned ex vivo studies using this technology have revealed significant morphological differences between healthy and cancerous tissue. However, the interpretation of MPM images by clinicians also remains a challenge and relies on their expertise in histopathology.

In contrast, OCT provides sub-surface structural information of the lesion under a label-free approach, with reported resolutions less than 10 μm and penetration capacities up to 2 mm. OCT can be used in combination with MPM, as both technologies provide complementary information useful for diagnosis assessment. While RCM and MPM 2D images are obtained horizontally in the transversal plane (also called "en-face"), OCT 2D images (B-scan) are obtained axially in depth in the coronal or sagittal plane. Furthermore, since OCT also allows obtaining 3D images (C-scan), lesions can be studied volumetrically from different points or axes of visualization. Although OCT images have less resolution than RCM and MPM images, the penetration capacity is higher, and the acquisition time is generally lower. This OCT aspect is of great importance to evaluate lesion margins and tumor infiltration into the mucosa under real-time situations in clinical environments.

OCT technology capabilities in the diagnosis of colon polyps have been investigated in the latest years with promising results on the future adoption in clinical practice. Several studies [18–21], both in murine and human models, have reported the identification of tissue layers and the discrimination capacities of the technology on the differentiation of different types of benign (including healthy) and malignant tissue. When analyzing 44 polyps from 24 patients [18], endoscopists detected fewer subsurface structures and a lower degree of light scattering in adenomas, and that, in comparison, hyperplastic polyps were closer in structure and light scattering to healthy mucosa. The scattering property was calculated by a computer program applying statistical analysis (Fisher–Freeman–Halton test and Spearman rank correlation test), confirming the previous appreciation. A comparison of OCT images with respect to histopathological images was performed in [19] using previously defined criteria for OCT image interpretation on the identification of tissue layers. Upon the observations, hyperplastic polyps are characterized by a three-layer structure (with mucosa thickening) whereas adenomas are characterized by the lack of layers. Then, under these assumptions, measured over a group of 116 polyps from patients, lesions could be visually differentiated in OCT images with 0.92 sensitivity and 0.84 specificity. Later, a fluorescence-guided study performed on 21 mice [20] after administrating a contrast agent showed the OCT ability to differentiate healthy mucosa, early dysplasia, and adenocarcinoma. Visual analysis of normal tissue revealed that the submucosa layer is very thin in some specimens and not always well appreciated in the OCT images, although the tissue boundaries remain distinguishable. In adenoma polyps, a thickening of the mucosa (in first stages) or disappearance of the boundary between layers is detected, whereas in the case of adenocarcinoma, the OCT images showed a loss of tissue texture, absence of layers, and the presence of dark spots caused by the high absorption in necrotic areas. In the latest study [21], they go beyond and propose a diagnosis criterion over micro OCT images with some similarities to the Kudo pit pattern [22] and demonstrate the diagnosis capacity of the OCT technology as clinicians can reach 0.9688 sensitivity and 0.9231 specificity on the identification of adenomas over 58 polyps from patients.

Both the cross sectional and the en-face images have been shown to provide clinically relevant information in the mentioned studies, and the combination of both views for the detailed study of tissue features suggests an important advance [23–25]. In addition to previous studies, the calculation of the angular spectrum of the scattering coefficient map has also revealed quantifiable variances on the different tissue types [26].

The clinical characteristics of the lesions that can be observed on the OCT images can be further exploited by image-based analysis. Image and signal processing methods can allow dealing with the noisy nature of the signal, whereas machine learning algorithms are able to exploit the spatial correlation of the biological structures to make the most of them. These types of algorithms can detect, and quantify, subtle variations on images that the naked human eye cannot and can be applied with the goal of performing automatic interpretation of the images for image enhancement, lesion delimitation, or classification tasks. However, as seen in previously reviewed studies, few attempts of applying these methods for colon polyps on OCT images have been found, showing that there are opportunities of research in the area.

The main limitation of traditional machine learning methods is the need to process the original data from their natural form to another form of representation appropriate for the targeted problem. Image processing methods must be carefully applied to extract the most representative features of the data, aiming to resemble how the experts analyze the images. Then, the extracted features are passed as input to the selected classifier method. Unlike deep learning approaches, traditional machine learning methods require tailored feature extraction which is followed by a shallow machine learning method. This makes them less prone to generalization and leads to lower discriminative power [27]. Under the deep learning paradigm, image feature extraction and classification are simultaneously performed through a network architecture representing all possible solution domains and which is optimized by means of a loss function minimization that seamlessly drives the network parameters towards a suitable solution. Convolutional neural networks (CNN) [28,29] have surpassed classical machine learning methods [30,31], and even medical expert capabilities [32–34]. They have been also successfully applied in colon cancer histopathological classification [35,36], MPM classification [37], polyp detection on colonoscopy [38–40], or histological colon tissue staining [41].

The application of deep learning methods to OCT medical images is a recent trend and only few examples of application are available. Ophthalmology being the oldest context of application of OCT, most examples are found in this area, and some others in cardiology and breast cancer [42–45]. In gastroenterology of the lower track (colon), only one recent work has been identified [46]. A pattern recognition network called RetinaNet [47] has been trained to distinguish normal from neoplastic tissue with a 1.0 sensitivity and 0.997 specificity. The success of the model is based on a dentate structural pattern, identified in normal tissue in previous studies, being utilized as a structural marker on the images used as input during training and evaluation. In this sense, the B-scan images on the dataset (26,000 images acquired from 20 tumor areas) are manually inspected to identify "teeth" samples representing normal colonic mucosa and "noisy" samples representing malignant tissue. On evaluation, the network provides a list of boxes where these patterns are found along with the probability, and average scores are calculated over a sequence of N adjacent B-scan images. The drawback of this approach resides in the identification of the "teeth" pattern in normal tissue, but no other patterns have been identified for malignant tissue, just assuming that the "teeth" pattern does not appear in that case.

The work presented in this paper further investigates the application of deep learning methods over a collected database with more than 94,000 OCT images of murine (rat) colon polyps to study the discrimination capacity of this imaging technique for its future adoption as a real-time optical biopsy method. The aim of this proposal is to contribute to setting the bases for the automatic analysis of images with latest state-of-the-art techniques that could lead to the development of new computer-aided diagnosis (CADx) applications. Once image analysis methods demonstrate this capacity, colon polyp diagnosis with OCT can be progressively mastered by clinicians and the adoption of the technology naturally accomplished. With this aim, this work implements a classification (benign vs. malignant) approach based on an Xception deep learning model that is trained and tested over a large dataset of OCT images from murine (rat) samples that have been collected for this purpose. We propose a pre-processing method for data augmentation and to validate the application of deep learning methods for colon polyp classification as benign or malignant. In addition, to further investigate the diagnosis capacity of the proposed approach, evaluation is performed twice, once over individual B-scan images and then also over C-scan volumes for comparison. Finally, a strategy to maximize results when evaluating individual B-scans is applied.

In comparison with previous studies [46], this work proposes a general diagnosis strategy based on classification instead of pattern recognition, which avoids time consuming manual annotation of the database providing automatic identification of the characteristics representing polyps tissue type. The classification strategy model can generalize better upon new polyp categories than the segmentation strategy, the performance of which is biased by the available annotations of the database. A classification strategy can help in the identification of subtle characteristics present on noisy OCT images that are not easily distinguished by the naked eye, and with proper visualization of them, can help clinicians to better understand the OCT imaging technique. In the future, the combination of both approaches could be considered for maximizing automatic diagnosis results.

2. Materials and Methods

2.1. Animal Models

Sixty animals with colorectal cancer (CRC) from the strain PIRC (polyposis in the rat colon) rat F344/NTac-Apcam1137 model (sex ratio: 50/50) from the Rat Resource and Research Centre (RRRC) were used for the extraction of neoplastic colonic samples. This animal model was used in the study for the following main reasons: (a) it is an excellent model for studying human familial colon cancer; (b) ENU (N-ethyl-N-nitrosourea)-induced point mutation results in a truncating mutation in the APC (adenomatous polyposis coli) gene at a site corresponding to the human mutation hotspot region of the gene; (c) heterozygotes develop multiple tumors in the small intestine and colon by 2–4 months of age; (d) PIRC tumors closely resemble those in humans in terms of histopathology and morphology as well as distribution between intestine and colon; (e) provides longer lifespan compared to related mouse models (10–15 months); and (f) tumors may be visualized by CT (computerized tomography), endoscopy, or dissection. Moreover, the absolute incidence and multiplicity of colonic tumors are higher in F344-PIRC rats than in carcinogen-treated wild-type F344 rats, or in mice [48,49].

Additionally, thirty rats from the strain Fischer344—F344 wildtype model (sex ratio: 50/50) were used for the development and extraction of hyperplastic colonic samples. A rat surgical model of hyperplasia in the colon was developed in novo for endoscopic applications. It recreates important features of human hyperplasia, such as the generation of new cells in the colonic mucosa and tissue growth, as well as the corresponding angiogenesis. It consists of an extracolonic suture on which lesions are inflicted with a biopsy extraction forceps during a period established in different weekly follow-ups for the correct induction of the model [50,51].

Finally, as a control group, ten healthy tissue samples from three specimens were extracted from the colon of rats from the strain Fischer344—F344 wildtype model (sex ratio: 50/50). Uninvolved areas of the hyperplasia animals (ascending colon, transverse colon, and regions of the descending colon without lesion) were used as healthy tissue samples. This ensured meeting one of the three r's of animal research that aims to maximize the information obtained per animal, making it possible to limit or avoid further use of other animals, without compromising animal welfare.

2.2. Equipment

The equipment used for imaging the murine (rat) samples was a CALLISTO from Thorlabs (CAL110C1) [52] spectral domain system with central wavelength 930 nm, field of view of 6 × 6 mm^2, 7 µm axial resolution, 4 µm lateral resolution, 1.7 mm measurement in depth, 107 dB sensitivity at 1.2 kHz measurement speed, and 7.5 mm working distance. Samples were scanned using the high-resolution scan lens (18 mm focal length) and a standard probe head with a rigid scanner for stable and easy-to-operate setup.

2.3. Acquisition Procedure

2.3.1. Sample Acquisition Procedure

Rats were acclimatized before surgery in individually housed cages at 22–25 °C with food and water ad libitum. All surgical procedures were performed under general inhalation anesthesia [53–55] by placing them in an induction chamber to administrate sevoflurane 6–8% in oxygen with a high flow of fresh gas (1 L/min). Then, they were connected to a face mask to continue the administration of sevoflurane (3–3.5%) in oxygen (300 mL/min) and placed in dorsal decubitus to carry out the endoscopic procedure. Atropine (0.05 mg/kg), meloxicam (1 mg/kg/24 h), and pethidine (10–20 mg/kg) were injected subcutaneously before beginning the surgical procedure. A thermal blanket was used throughout the procedure. Once the animals had acquired the appropriate surgical plane, a colonoscopy was performed to rule out the presence of abnormalities that could interfere with the study. The aim was locating all those lesions that could be found through observation by using white light and a rigid cystourethroscope of 2.9 mm in diameter, which reached a diameter of up to 5 mm when working with an intermediate sheath and an external sheath (size appropriate for this animal model), with the objective of not damaging said structures at the start of the procedure. After shaving the abdomen and preparing the area with povidone-iodine and 70% ethanol, animals were covered with an open sterile cloth. Then, an average laparotomy of 4–5 cm in length was performed. A retraction device with hooks (Lonestar®) was used as support tool to make this section circular and externalize all the necessary intestinal content outside the abdomen. Animals were kept at constant temperature thanks to successive peritoneal washes made with tempered serum. Then, the block of the colon was fixated with a suture to prevent the reversion of the content throughout the colon and cecum. Three areas (ascending colon, transverse colon, and descending colon) were studied consecutively taking advantage of the anatomical division of the colon. They were divided with the help of ligatures (silk 4/0) through the mesentery of each portion and scanned in the proximal to distal direction making use of the rigid cystoscope to check the number of polyps.

At each point with lesions, a disposable bulldog clamp was used to mark the distribution of the lesions, thus avoiding cutting the lesions in the next procedure of colostomy of ascending and transverse portions. After that, the colon was extracted in block and then, the animals were euthanized under general inhalation anesthesia by rapid intracardiac injection of potassium chloride (KCl) (2 mEq/kg, KCl 2M), according to the ethical committee recommendations. The colon was opened by a longitudinal colotomy with the help of scissors to eliminate the tube shape of the colon, exposing thus the mucosa with the localized polyps to improve their visualization, handling, and analysis. At this time, magnification was provided by a STORZ VITOM® HD for a better location of the lesions with the extended organ.

For each localized lesion, a sample was extracted for later ex vivo analysis with the OCT equipment. Instead of acquiring the images directly on the fresh sample after resection, samples were fixed and then preserved for several further analyses while maintaining the properties of the tissue. Based on [56], the fixation procedure for each sample consisted in the immersion of the sample in 4% formaldehyde for at least 14 h at about 4 °C. Then, after two washes with phosphate buffered saline 0.01 M (PBS) each 30 min, the sample was submerged in PBS and 0.1% of sodium azide and stored in refrigeration at 4 °C. This method was established to provide safer handling of samples, avoiding the adverse effects of manipulating formaldehyde-embedded samples in a surgical environment. Additionally, it was checked with histopathological analysis that this fixation procedure did not alter the properties of the tissue, showing no noticeable differences from fresh tissue.

2.3.2. Image Acquisition Protocol

First, each sample was placed on a plate, secured, and fixed for the correct exposure of the tissue. Once placed on the platform under the OCT probe, a B-scan of the sample was acquired for further calibration of the equipment. While scanning, the sample was focused by approaching the OCT probe. The super-fine focus allows to acquire a high-quality OCT signal with the better penetration depth. Due to the anatomical differences of the samples, it was always necessary to repeat this step for each new sample. Once the sample was properly focused and the 2D signal quality optimized, the next step was the acquisition of a C-scan of the sample. In this case, the software allowed drawing a rectangle (Figure 1) indicating where to perform the 3D acquisition on the sample. When considered, various 3D scans covering different parts of the lesion were recorded for the same lesion.

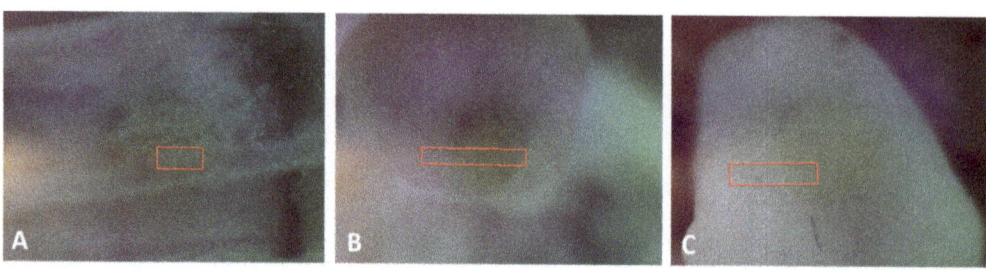

Figure 1. Pre-view of tissue/lesions with C-scan scanning area selected in red. (**A**): healthy sample; (**B**): neoplastic polyp 1; (**C**): neoplastic polyp 2.

2.3.3. Dataset Summary

The database consists of healthy, hyperplastic, and neoplastic (adenomatous and adenocarcinoma) samples. Following the previously described acquisition procedure, the subsequent number of cases were included in the database for each tissue type: 10 healthy samples with 48 C-scans, 13 hyperplastic samples with 53 C-scans, and 75 neoplastic samples with 245 C-scans. As a result, the database contains a total of 94,687 B-scan images.

The database was visually inspected before training the model ignoring all C-scans or B-scan images acquired with errors, large aberrations, or artifacts to ensure the quality of the data. Note that this database is a preliminary version of an ongoing larger dataset that will be made openly available. Access to the database used in this article is possible upon request to the corresponding author.

2.4. Ethical Considerations

Ethical approvals for murine (rat) samples acquisition were obtained from the relevant Ethics Committees. In case of research with animals, it was approved by the Ethical Committee of animal experimentation of the Jesús Usón Minimally Invasive Surgery Centre (Number: ES 100370001499) and was in accordance with the welfare standards of the regional government which are based on European regulations.

2.5. Deep Learning Architecture

The proposed architecture was based on the Xception classification model [57] previously trained over the ImageNet dataset [58]. Then, a global average pooling layer and a final layer with 2 neurons and softmax activation were added, representing the classification classes: benign vs. malignant. A schematic view of the architecture, generated with a visual grammar tool [59], is provided in Figure 2.

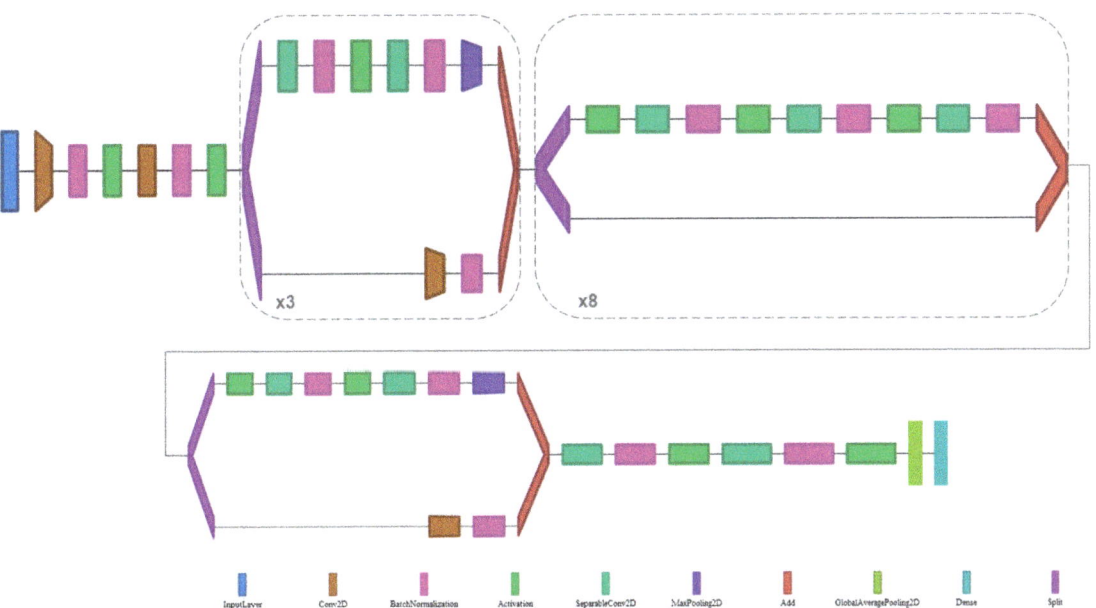

Figure 2. Schematic diagram of deep learning architecture based on the Xception model.

This pre-trained network accepts images of the size of 299 × 299 pixels which are randomly sampled from the original OCT images as detailed in next section "data preparation and augmentation". OCT images on the database (B-scan images) have variable lateral sizes in the range 512–2000 pixels due to differences in the sizes of the polyps and scanning area selected. For this reason, B-scan images were pre-processed to extract regions of interest of smaller size (299 × 299 pixels) to make the most of the images and avoid losing lesion structural features on the bigger images that would happen with image rescaling. Directly rescaling the whole image could be comparable to reducing the lateral and axial resolution of the images, and hence losing information about the smaller structures. The proposed data preparation approach also serves as a data augmentation strategy. Moreover, a strategy for dealing with data imbalance in the dataset was also adopted.

2.5.1. Data Preparation and Augmentation

As a data augmentation strategy, during the training process, the algorithm processes the dataset images in the following manner: image pre-processing; air-tissue delimitation; random selection of region of interest (ROI); ROI extraction; and ROI preparation. These steps are illustrated in Figure 3.

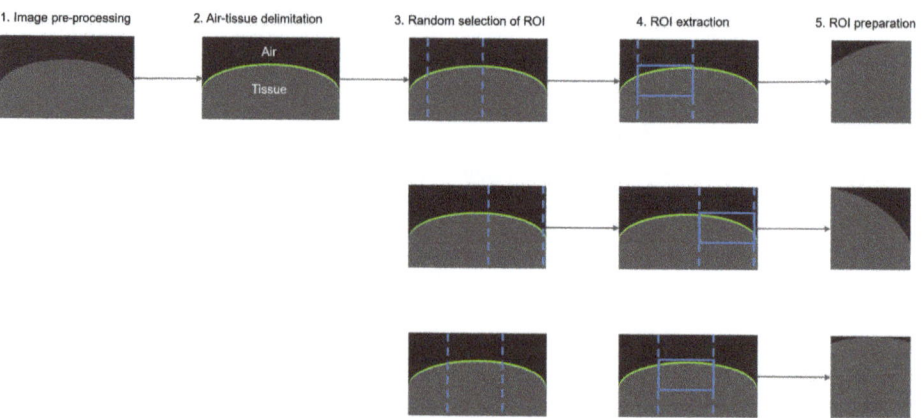

Figure 3. Proposed image data preparation methodology. 1. Image pre-processing, 2. air-tissue delimitation, 3. random selection of region of interest (ROI), 4. ROI extraction, and 5. ROI preparation.

1. Image pre-processing

    The OCT gray scale original image contains one single channel that is duplicated to generate the 3-channel image expected by the network to use the ImageNet pre-trained weights. As an additional data augmentation strategy, the image is randomly flipped horizontally to produce alternative input images. No additional geometric transformations are applied to the image, as this would alter the structural features of the lesion and lead to misclassification.

2. Air-tissue delimitation

    The aim of this step is to automatically detect on the image the delimitation between the air and the tissue. The final goal of this operation is to obtain ROI images adjusted to the tissue, so the noise present in the air part and the differences on the distance from the scanning tip to the tissue in the database images do not provide ambiguous information to the network. Conversely, the shape of the lesion is preserved, and flattering is discarded, as this could be a clinically interesting feature for differentiating the lesion's diagnostic nature.

    This step was implemented following the next sub-steps: automatic calculation of Otsu threshold [60] to differentiate between the air and the tissue regions; binary mask generation applying the calculated Otsu threshold to the image; morphological operation to remove small objects from the binary mask; then, for each column in the mask image, extraction of the location (row) of the first positive (true) value if available, to obtain a 1D array containing the delimitation path; and application of a median filter (kernel size = 69) to the delimitation array to eliminate or smooth possible noise in the signal.

3. Random selection of region of interest

Considering that the total width of the input image (number of A-scans) is highly variable for the different images of the dataset due to the sample size and scanning conditions, a random number indicating where to start the region of interest is calculated. A preliminary sub-image (column) is obtained considering a width of 512 px for the region of interest.

4. ROI extraction

The values of the delimitation array are applied to the previously extracted sub-image to adjust the tissue at the top, generating a ROI of 512 px width and 224 px depth, which is equivalent to approximately 0.71 mm in width and 0.75 mm in depth considering the optics of the device. Preliminary experiments with fewer widths or longer depths reported worse results. Smaller ROIs reduce the maintained information worsening the feature extraction and classification performance, so it is important to reach an agreement between both aspects.

5. ROI preparation (post-processing)

The extracted ROIs are resized to 229 px width and 299 px depth to match the default input size of the network (pre-trained with ImageNet).

2.5.2. Data Imbalance Management

This work aims at differentiating benign samples, including healthy tissue and hyperplastic polyps, from malignant/neoplastic samples, including adenomatous and adenocarcinomatous samples. Unfortunately, in our dataset, healthy and hyperplastic samples are underrepresented with respect to neoplastic samples. Data imbalance is a usual problem and for the moment there is not a best strategy for dealing with it, as it mostly depends on the problem to solve and on data characteristics. In this work, a resampling strategy was implemented. This strategy was preferred to weight balance compensation, where weights of each class are calculated and specified on network fitting, as in the authors' experience, it provides better results.

Resampling is a classical strategy for dealing with data imbalance. Over-sampling means adding more samples to the minority class, whereas under-sampling means removing samples for the majority class. Over-sampling and under-sampling can be achieved following different strategies, with the weakness that these may imply. The simplest way is to randomly duplicate or remove samples.

In this work, we implemented an over-sampling strategy by adding new samples for the minority class. However, these new samples were not exact copies of original data, as small variations were introduced to create a diverse set of samples. As described in the previous section, dataset images were manipulated for randomly obtaining ROIs (see Figure 3), that in addition were randomly horizontally flipped, which allowed introducing this variability in the training and validation set.

2.5.3. Training Process

The implemented network was based on a Xception model [57], where a global average pooling layer followed by a dense layer (with two outputs and softmax activation) to deal with a 2-class problem (benign vs. malignant) was added at the end. Pre-trained weights of ImageNet were used [58].

Categorical cross entropy loss was minimized by an Adam optimizer with a learning rate of 0.0001 during the training process. The selected batch size is 24, for a number of 100 epochs and validation loss minimization was monitored for early stopping (with patience 20). The training process was repeated 6 times over different data splits to make sure that the provided results were not biased.

2.5.4. Data Evaluation and Test-Time Augmentation

As described before, OCT C-scans were acquired from murine (rat) polyp samples and adjacent healthy tissue. The C-scans are 3D volumes that consist of consecutive and adjacent B-scan images. For some of the polyps, several C-scans covering different parts of the lesion (upper, center, and bottom) were obtained and included in the same data split. As one of the aims of this work was to study the diagnosis capacity and limitations of OCT in more detail, the evaluation of the model was designed with the intention of comparing the discrimination capacity of the individual B-scans classification with respect to C-scans.

A test time augmentation (TTA) strategy was applied to B-scan and C-scan evaluation. This was implemented by performing 10 augmentations over the data following the random ROI extraction strategy previously described (see Figure 3) and then calculating the mean prediction. By applying this strategy, we estimated a richer posterior probability distribution function of the prediction for the bigger (wider) B-scans. We present a comparison of the results without TTA (called standard) and with TTA to facilitate studying how this technique contributed to the proposed approach.

3. Results

3.1. OCT and H&E Histology Comparative Analysis

Before performing the analysis, it was important to consider that some anatomical differences exist between human colon and murine colon structure. According to [61], in human and rats species, the colon maintains the same mural structure as the rest of the gastrointestinal tract: mucosa, submucosa, and inner circular and outer longitudinal tunica muscularis and serosa. The mucosa and submucosa layers in mice are relative thin in comparison with the human ones. Furthermore, human mucosa has transverse folds through the entire colon, whereas in mice it varies for each part of the colon. At the cecum and proximal colon, mouse mucosa has transverse folds, in the mid colon is flat, and in the distal colon has longitudinal folds. However, in both species the mucosa is composed of tubular glands. Taking this into account and considering that the database used in this work consists of murine (rat) samples, it was expected that the model also learn these anatomical differences present in the mucosa, especially for the healthy samples. A detailed comparison of the anatomical differences (extracted from reference [61]) is provided in Table A1.

According to previous studies analyzing features on OCT images [18–21], in normal tissue, well-defined layers can be visualized with uniform intensity. In the presence of hyperplasia, thickening of the mucosa layer occurs, but the intensity is similar to healthy tissue and tissue layers are still visible. However, in the case of adenomatous polyps, both thickening of the mucosa and reduced intensity must be observed. Finally, adenocarcinomatous lesions should show blurred boundaries and non-uniform intensity. In the presence of large polyps, the disappearance of the boundaries should be clearly observed, independently from the lesion nature.

Visual inspection of dataset images was performed to look for the features previously mentioned. Figures 4 and 5 provide a detailed analysis of the visible features on the OCT images (of Figure 1 samples) with respect to the histopathological hematoxylin-eosin (H&E) images annotated by a pathologist (scanned at 5x). Regions of interest (with the same FOV of OCT images in mm) were extracted from H&E slides images and later rescaled to fit axial and lateral resolution of the OCT images for better comparison. In these figures, it can be observed that the main features present in H&E images can also be observed in the OCT images. On the one hand, Figure 4, representing healthy tissue, illustrates (as indicated by arrows and manual segmentation lines on the B-scans on the left, Figure 4A,B) that the mucosa layers can be very clearly observed, confirming what has been reported before in previous studies. Muscularis mucosae and sub-mucosa layers are also observed, although clear differentiation in all parts of the image is tougher. On the other side, when analyzing Figure 5 containing neoplastic lesions, it is also possible to confirm that the boundaries of the layers have totally disappeared, making it impossible to find any difference among them. Differences in the noise pattern are also observed. In addition, as indicated using circles and arrows on the B-scans (Figure 5A,B), new underlying structures appeared in the mucosa and can be identified as bright spots or dark areas in the images. These new structures (in comparison with healthy tissue) are also clearly observed in the corresponding annotated histopathology images (Figure 5C,D), where cystic crypts (CC) have been identified by the pathologist and appear as dark spots in the B-scan and tumoral glands (TG) clusters as bright spots.

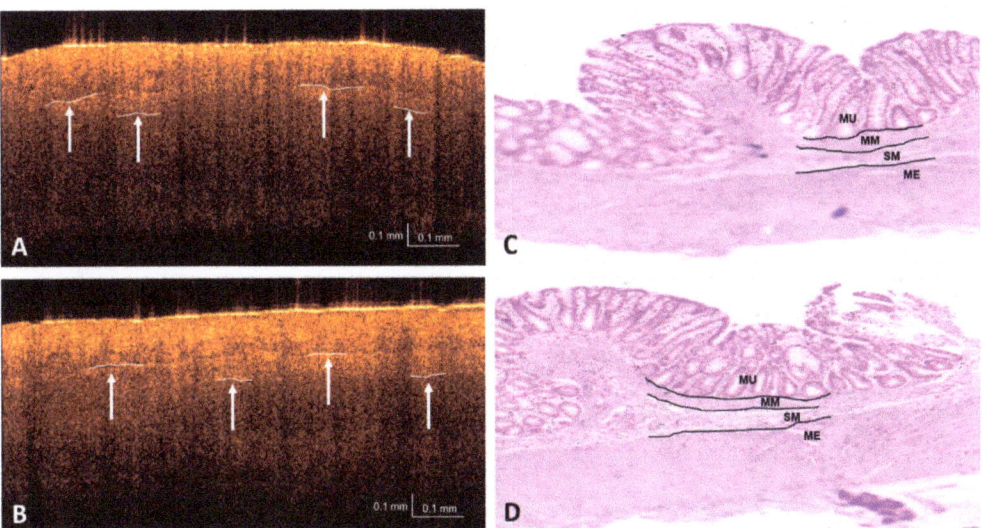

Figure 4. Comparison of features identified in optical coherence tomography (OCT) images (**A,B**) with respect to pathologists' annotations on H&E images (**C,D**) on healthy sample (Figure 1A). MU: mucosa, MM: muscularis mucosae, SM: submucosa, ME: muscularis externa.

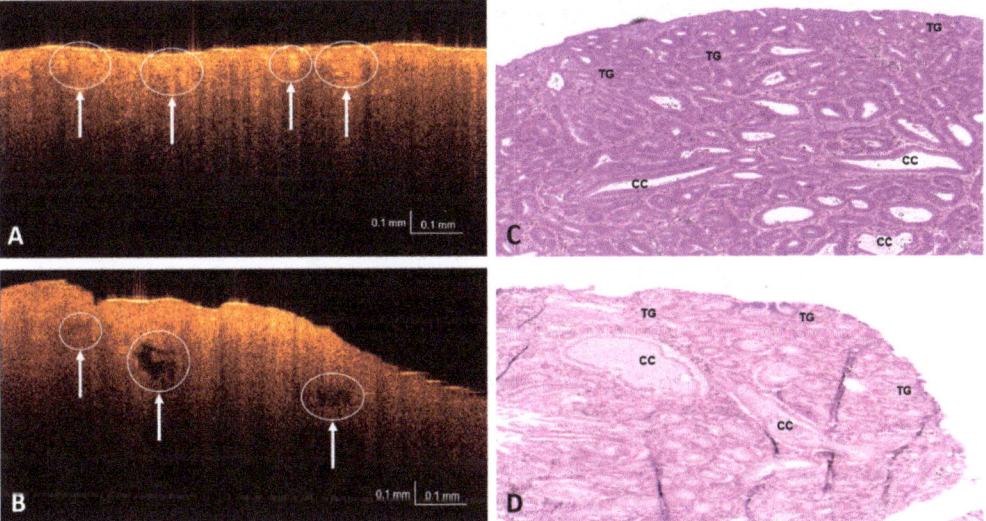

Figure 5. Comparison of features identified in OCT images (**A,B**) with respect to pathologists' annotations on H&E images (**C,D**) on neoplastic samples (Figure 1B,C). CC: cystic crypt, TG: tumoral glands.

3.2. Dataset Partitioning and Testing

The dataset was split such that 80% was dedicated to training, 10% to validation, and 10% to testing. It was assured that images coming from the same lesion (both B-scans and C-scans) were included in only one of the sets. The animal models employed on the creation of the database were genetically modified replicas of one specimen, hence no separation per specimen was necessary in splitting and lesions could be considered independently.

The model was tested on 6 different folds to ensure that the evaluation metrics proportionated were not biased by one random dataset split. A random state seed parameter was established for each fold to obtain different training, validation, and testing sets each time.

3.3. Performance Metrics and Evaluation

Given that both B-scan and C-scan data were available for the murine (rat) samples acquired in the database, the clinical discrimination capability of the model on the differentiation of benign versus malignant polyps was calculated for both types of data. To evaluate each C-scan, the mean of the individual predictions for the B-scan images that form the volume was calculated. The performance of the model was measured using the conditions provided by the confusion matrix (see Table 1).

Table 1. Confusion matrix conditions for metrics calculation.

		Actual Condition	
		Malignant	Benign
Predicted Condition	Malignant	TP	FP
	Benign	FN	TN

In the clinical context being analyzed in this work, these conditions can be seen as:

- True positive (TP): Malignant lesion correctly identified as malignant.
- False positive (FP): Benign lesion incorrectly identified as malignant.
- True negative (TN): Benign lesion correctly identified as benign.
- False negative (FN): Malignant lesion incorrectly identified as benign.

The metrics that were employed to measure the model performance based on the previous conditions are described below.

- Sensitivity. Also known as the true positive rate (TPR). Number of true/all positive assessments. TPR = TP/(TP + FN) = number of malign lesions with positive test/total number of malign lesions.
- Specificity. Also known as the true negative rate (TNR). Number of true/all negative assessments. TNR = TN/(FP + TN) = number of benign lesions with negative test/total number of benign lesions.
- Positive predictive value (PPV). In case of a malignant prediction, probability that the lesion is actually malignant. PPV = TP/(TP + FP) = Number of true positives/number of positive calls.
- Negative predictive value (NPV). In case of a benign prediction, probability that the lesion is actually benign. NPV = TN/(TN + FN) = Number of true negatives/number of negative calls.

The desired value for these metrics was as close as possible to 1, 1 meaning a perfect test.

Additionally, as the accuracy (measure of the number of samples that were correctly classified in the expected class) is a misleading metric in imbalanced datasets, the balanced accuracy was calculated. This metric normalizes true positive and true negative predictions by the number of positive and negative samples, and then divides the sum by two, providing an accuracy value where the class frequencies are the same.

- Balanced accuracy (BAC). Measures the number of samples that were correctly classified in the expected class considering class frequencies. Number of correct/all assessments considering class frequencies. BAC = (TPR + TNR)/2 = (Sensitivity + Specificity)/2.

3.4. Thresholds

Considering the prediction values provided by the model, the threshold that maximizes the BAC (in the range 0–1) was calculated over the validation subset of each fold split both for the B-scan and C-scan data. Then, this threshold was applied over the test subset of each fold split to calculate the metrics of the model (BAC, sensitivity, specificity, PPV, and NPV).

3.5. Classification Results

The evaluation of the model was performed on 6 folds, over different training, validation, and testing splits of the dataset each time, with the aim of obtaining a model ensemble. As a result, the mean and standard deviation (std) were calculated for each of the selected metrics. Table 2 provides a summary of the results, where the first number reports the mean and the second the std (mean ± std). In this summary, the results obtained with B-scan and C-scan images, standard, and TTA test split evaluation are included for comparison. The complete list of results of each fold is included in Table A2. at the end of the document. Additionally, a graph illustrating a fair comparison of the folds results following the sum of ranking differences (SRDs) method [62] is provided in Figure A1. After calculating the SRD coefficients for each of the options on the different folds, a graph comparing the performance of the different options can be generated. The smaller the SRD value, the closer to the reference value, meaning better performance.

Table 2. Summary of results by the network for the different imaging modalities (B-scan vs. C-scan), applying different evaluation techniques (standard vs. test time augmentation (TTA)) and resampling imbalance strategy. Note that the numbers report "mean ± std" values.

Data Type	Evaluation	BAC	Sensitivity	Specificity	PPV	NPV
B-scan	Standard	0.8806 ± 0.0748	0.9635 ± 0.0148	0.7978 ± 0.1431	0.9268 ± 0.0498	0.8914 ± 0.0415
	TTA	0.8895 ± 0.0792	0.8094 ± 0.1524	0.8094 ± 0.1524	0.9305 ± 0.0526	0.9093 ± 0.0400
C-scan	Standard	0.8857 ± 0.1143	0.7893 ± 0.2180	0.7893 ± 0.2180	0.9221 ± 0.0735	0.9432 ± 0.0687
	TTA	0.8843 ± 0.1068	0.7865 ± 0.2050	0.7865 ± 0.2050	0.9212 ± 0.0693	0.9472 ± 0.0614

4. Discussion and Conclusions

On analyzing the results, in general terms and considering the mean results reported in Table 2, when using the standard evaluation technique, the prediction over C-scan volumes was slightly better than the prediction over individual B-scan images. This impression is confirmed by the SRD analysis (Figure A1), where smaller values were obtained for C-scan images analysis. This result makes sense, since when evaluating the lesion volumetrically (C-scan) considering the mean prediction of all the B-scan images contained in the C-scan, there was less probability of a bad prediction. If the volume contains some individual B-scans with poor information representing the class sample, the (expected) bad predictions do not have great influence on the final diagnosis. In any case, the small differences on the prediction metrics suggest the high quality of the database used in this study, as shown in the detailed results for each fold provided in Table A2.

It can also be observed that the TTA evaluation technique slightly benefitted the prediction over individual B-scan images in terms of sensitivity and specificity, but not the C-scan volume prediction. However, these results make sense for two reasons: the data preparation strategy and the volumetric evaluation of the lesion. On the one hand, due to the nature of the images, no geometrical transformations were applied for data augmentation, as described in the data preparation section, but ROIs at different location of the image were extracted. Depending on the location of the extracted ROIs, the clinical features can be more or less representative of the lesion, affecting the corresponding prediction. When TTA was applied, different ROIs from the B-scan were extracted, allowing analysis of the overall sample in width, and hence a better prediction was obtained. This is particularly beneficial in the case of large wide B-scan images, as it allows analyzing the different parts of the tissue/lesion in detail. Considering this, and although no improvement was observed on the C-scan evaluation, the TTA strategy was preferred during the evaluation, since in this way, the intrinsic clinical variability of the lesions was captured and hence the model prediction was more robust.

Interpretation of new imaging techniques, such as OCT, can be complicated at the beginning and prevent their adoption in clinical practice. However, advanced image processing techniques, such as deep learning, can be used to facilitate automatic image analysis or diagnosis and the development of optical biopsy. A previous work [46] proposed using a pattern recognition network that requires prior manual annotation of the dataset and diagnosis depends on whether the expected pattern is found on the image. Alternatively, this work proposes using a classification strategy, which can help in the identification of subtle clinical characteristics on the images and is not biased by dataset annotations. This work investigates the application of an Xception deep learning model for the automatic classification of colon polyps from murine (rat) samples acquired with OCT imaging. The developed database is accessible upon request and is part of a bigger database in the process of being published. A strategy for processing B-scan images and extracting regions of interest was proposed as a data augmentation strategy. Test time augmentation strategy implemented with the aim of improving model prediction was evaluated. In addition, this work also aims to compare the differences in the diagnosis capacity of the proposed method when evaluated using B-scan images and C-scan volumes, and for this purpose different clinical metrics were compared. The trained model was evaluated 6 times using different training, validation, and testing sets to provide an unbiased diagnosis of the results. In this sense, we got a model with mean 0.9695 ($\pm$0.0141) sensitivity and mean 0.8094 ($\pm$0.1524) specificity when diagnosis was performed over individual B-scans, and mean 0.9821 ($\pm$0.0197) sensitivity and mean 0.7865 ($\pm$0.205) specificity when diagnosis was performed in the whole C-scan volume.

Considering the future application of a deep learning method to assist clinical diagnosis with OCT, and in view of the results of this work, successful diagnosis can be achieved both on B-scan images and C-scan volumes. The evaluation of the lesion over a C-scan volume was preferred over the evaluation of an individual B-scan image, so the prediction could be more robust. However, this will not be possible most of the time in the daily clinical routine, for example during patient colonoscopy examination, where in vivo real-time information is necessary for diagnosis and in-situ treatment decision. In this sense, clinical procedures based on the accumulative predictions of various B-scan images could be defined to facilitate clinicians' decision-making during examination. The promising results with the proposed approach suggest that the implemented deep learning based method can identify the clinical features reported in previous clinical studies on the OCT images, and more importantly, that the amount of data and features present on the images database are enough to allow automatic classification. These results are part of ongoing work that will be further extended; however, it has been demonstrated that deep learning-based strategies seem to be the path to achieve the "optical biopsy" paradigm. Raw interpretation of new imaging modalities is difficult for clinicians but assisted by an image analysis method, the interpretation can be eased and the reliable diagnosis suggestion can facilitate the adoption of the technology. Consequently, the CADx market can benefit from this progress in the short term as the latest market forecast studies suggest.

This work will be further extended and tested with a larger and more balanced version of the murine dataset collected. More sophisticated models accepting larger image size will be tested to check whether classification is improved. Optical properties of the different lesions will be studied in detail with the aim of finding scattering patterns for each type of lesion. OCT volumetric (C-scan) information will be also studied in further detail to make the most of it analyzing both the cross sectional and en-face views.

Author Contributions: Conceptualization, C.L.S., J.B., and J.F.O.-M.; methodology, C.L.S., A.P., and E.T.; software, C.L.S.; validation, C.L.S., J.B., N.A.d.R., and N.A.; formal analysis, C.L.S., A.P., and E.T.; investigation, C.L.S.; resources, J.B., J.F.O.-M., E.G., O.M.C., N.A.d.R., and N.A.; data curation, C.L.S., J.B., J.F.O.-M., N.A.d.R., and N.A.; writing—original draft preparation, C.L.S., J.B., and J.F.O.-M.; writing—review and editing, C.L.S., J.B., J.F.O.-M., A.P., E.T., E.G., and O.M.C.; visualization, C.L.S.; supervision, E.G. and O.M.C.; project administration, C.L.S., A.P., and E.G.; funding acquisition, C.L.S. and A.P. All authors have read and agreed to the published version of the manuscript.

Funding: This work was partially supported by PICCOLO project. This project has received funding from the European Union's Horizon2020 Research and Innovation Programme under grant agreement No. 732111. The sole responsibility of this publication lies with the authors. The European Union is not responsible for any use that may be made of the information contained therein. This research has also received funding from the Basque Government's Industry Department under the ELKARTEK program's project ONKOTOOLS under agreement KK-2020/00069 and the industrial doctorate program UC- DI14 of the University of Cantabria.

Institutional Review Board Statement: Ethical approvals for murine (rat) samples acquisition were obtained from the relevant Ethics Committees. In case of research with animals, it was approved by the Ethical Committee of animal experimentation of the Jesús Usón Minimally Invasive Surgery Centre (Number: ES 100370001499) and was in accordance with the welfare standards of the regional government which are based on European regulations.

Informed Consent Statement: Not applicable.

Data Availability Statement: The dataset used in this study is available upon request. This dataset is part of a more extensive dataset that is under collection and will be made publicly available in the future.

Acknowledgments: The authors would also like to thank Ainara Egia Bizkarralegorra from Basurto University hospital (Spain) for the processing of the samples.

Conflicts of Interest: The authors declare no conflict of interest. The funders had no role in the design of the study; in the collection, analyses, or interpretation of data; in the writing of the manuscript, or in the decision to publish the results.

Appendix A

Table A1. Comparison of anatomical differences of human and murine colon (adapted from reference [61]).

Feature	Human	Rats
Anatomy of the large intestine compared macroscopically		
Cecum to rectum	~100–150 cm	~25 cm
Taenia coli and haustra	Present	None; smooth serosa; may have fecal pellets
Appendix	Present, vermiform, ~9 cm	Absent
Functional cecum	Absent	Present; fermentation, vitamins K and B
Proximal/ascending/right	Colon from ileocecal valve to the hepatic flexure	Transverse folds in the mucosa, from cecum to mid colon; Rat: folds are visible through serosa
Mid/transverse	Connects the hepatic to the splenic flexure	Very short; lumen narrows; no mucosal folds
Distal/descending/left	Splenic flexure to left lower quadrant; S-shaped sigmoid colon extends from descending colon to rectosigmoid junction; sigmoid colon may be redundant	Fecal pellets may be seen
Rectum	12–15 cm curved; proximal two-thirds of rectum has a mesothelial covering within the peritoneal cavity, whereas the distal third of rectum is extraperitoneal, lying within the deep pelvis, surrounded by adventitia, fascia, and fat	Indistinct from distal colon; Rat: ~50–80 mm, prolapse is rare
Large intestine anatomy compared at histological level		
Mucosa	Transverse folds at all regions	Mucosal folds vary by region. Cecum and proximal colon: transverse; mid colon: flat with no folds; distal colon and rectum: longitudinal
Absorptive colonocytes	Similar to rodent	Present
Mucous/goblet cells	Similar to rodent	Present
Enteroendocrine cells	Similar to rodent	Present
Paneth cells	Cecum and appendix	Absent
Microfold (M) cells	Similar to rodent	Present
Lamina propria	Similar to rodent	Lymphocytes, plasma cells, macrophages, eosinophils, mast cells
Muscularis mucosae	Variable thickness; traversed by lymphoid follicles; poorly developed in appendix	Thin
Submucosa	Contains adipose tissue, arterioles, venules, lymphatics, and Meissner's plexus	Rodents thinner than humans
Muscular tunics	Auerbach's plexus between the two muscle bands	Muscular tunics thicken distally
Proximal colon	Transverse folds	Transverse mucosal folds
Transverse colon	Transverse folds	Flat mucosa
Distal colon	Transverse folds	Longitudinal mucosal folds
Rectum	Transverse folds	Indistinguishable from distal colon

Appendix B

Table A2. Detail of the results of each fold for the different imaging modalities (B-scan vs. C-scans).

Fold	Data Type	Evaluation	BAC	Sensitivity	Specificity	PPV	NPV
1	B-scan	Standard	0.8967	0.9472	0.8462	0.9207	0.8948
		TTA	0.9024	0.9553	0.8494	0.9229	0.9098
	C-scan	Standard	0.8736	0.9615	0.7857	0.8929	0.9167
		TTA	0.8736	0.9615	0.7857	0.8929	0.9167
2	B-scan	Standard	0.9000	0.9583	0.8417	0.9362	0.8928
		TTA	0.9060	0.9616	0.8505	0.9398	0.9012
	C-scan	Standard	0.8988	0.9643	0.8333	0.9310	0.9091
		TTA	0.8988	0.9643	0.8333	0.9310	0.9091
3	B-scan	Standard	0.7568	0.9549	0.5588	0.8455	0.8305
		TTA	0.7590	0.9585	0.5594	0.8461	0.8421
	C-scan	Standard	0.6917	0.9667	0.4167	0.8056	0.8333
		TTA	0.7333	0.9667	0.5000	0.8286	0.8571
4	B-scan	Standard	0.8311	0.9657	0.6966	0.9037	0.8732
		TTA	0.8398	0.9790	0.7007	0.9048	0.9189
	C-scan	Standard	0.8500	1.0000	0.7000	0.9032	1.0000
		TTA	0.8000	1.0000	0.6000	0.8750	1.0000
5	B-scan	Standard	0.9437	0.9642	0.9233	0.9733	0.8988
		TTA	0.9587	0.9705	0.9468	0.9815	0.9172
	C-scan	Standard	1.0000	1.0000	1.0000	1.0000	1.0000
		TTA	1.0000	1.0000	1.0000	1.0000	1.0000
6	B-scan	Standard	0.9553	0.9905	0.9201	0.9812	0.9584
		TTA	0.9709	0.9922	0.9495	0.9881	0.9666
	C-scan	Standard	1.0000	1.0000	1.0000	1.0000	1.0000
		TTA	1.0000	1.0000	1.0000	1.0000	1.0000

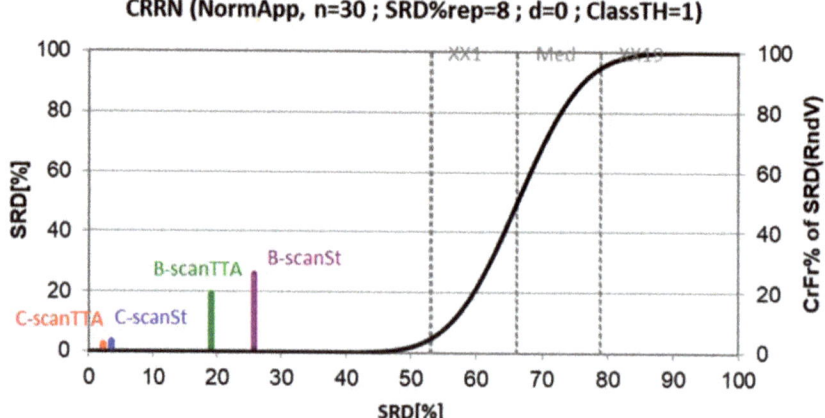

Figure A1. Fair comparison of folds results with sum of ranking differences (SRDs) method.

References

1. Office World Health Organization Europe. Colorectal Cancer. Available online: https://www.euro.who.int/en/health-topics/noncommunicable-diseases/cancer/news/news/2012/2/early-detection-of-common-cancers/colorectal-cancer (accessed on 15 December 2020).
2. World Cancer Research Fund International. Colorectal Cancer Statistics. Available online: https://www.wcrf.org/dietandcancer/cancer-trends/colorectal-cancer-statistics, (accessed on 15 December 2020).
3. Society, A.C. Can Colorectal Polyps and Cancer Be Found Early? Available online: https://www.cancer.org/cancer/colon-rectal-cancer/detection-diagnosis-staging/detection.html (accessed on 15 December 2020).
4. Axon, A.; Diebold, M.D.; Fujino, M.; Fujita, R.; Genta, R.M.; Gonvers, J.J.; Guelrud, M.; Inoue, H.; Jung, M.; Kashida, H.; et al. Update on the Paris classification of superficial neoplastic lesions in the digestive tract. *Endoscopy* **2005**, *37*, 570–578.
5. Hewett, D.G.; Kaltenbach, T.; Sano, Y.; Tanaka, S.; Saunders, B.P.; Ponchon, T.; Soetikno, R.; Rex, D.K. Validation of a simple classification system for endoscopic diagnosis of small colorectal polyps using narrow-band imaging. *Gastroenterology* **2012**, *143*, 599–607. [CrossRef]
6. Kavic, S.M.; Basson, M.D. Complications of endoscopy. *Am. J. Surg.* **2001**, *181*, 319–332. [CrossRef]
7. Reumkens, A.; Rondagh, E.J.A.; Bakker, C.M.; Winkens, B.; Masclee, A.A.M.; Sanduleanu, S. Post-colonoscopy complications: A systematic review, time trends, and meta-analysis of population-based studies. *Am. J. Gastroenterol.* **2016**, *111*, 1092–1101. [CrossRef] [PubMed]
8. Kandel, P.; Wallace, M.B. Should we resect and discard low risk diminutive colon polyps. *Clin. Endosc.* **2019**, *52*, 239–246. [CrossRef] [PubMed]
9. Glover, B.; Teare, J.; Patel, N. The Status of Advanced Imaging Techniques for Optical Biopsy of Colonic Polyps. *Clin. Transl. Gastroenterol.* **2020**, *11*, e00130. [CrossRef] [PubMed]
10. Levine, A.; Markowitz, O. Introduction to reflectance confocal microscopy and its use in clinical practice. *JAAD Case Rep.* **2018**, *4*, 1014–1023. [CrossRef] [PubMed]
11. Zhao, Y.; Iftimia, N.V. Overview of supercontinuum sources for multiphoton microscopy and optical biopsy. In *Neurophotonics and Biomedical Spectroscopy*; Elsevier: Amsterdam, The Netherlands, 2018; pp. 329–351.
12. Drexler, W.; Fujimoto, J.G. *Optical Coherence Tomography-Technology and Applications*; Springer: Berlin/Heidelberg, Germany, 2008.
13. Mason, S.E.; Poynter, L.; Takats, Z.; Darzi, A.; Kinross, J.M. Optical Technologies for Endoscopic Real-Time Histologic Assessment of Colorectal Polyps: A Meta-Analysis. *Am. J. Gastroenterol.* **2019**, *114*, 1219–1230. [CrossRef]
14. Taunk, P.; Atkinson, C.D.; Lichtenstein, D.; Rodriguez-Diaz, E.; Singh, S.K. Computer-assisted assessment of colonic polyp histopathology using probe-based confocal laser endomicroscopy. *Int. J. Colorectal Dis.* **2019**, *34*, 2043–2051. [CrossRef]
15. Ussui, V.M.; Wallace, M.B. Confocal endomicroscopy of colorectal polyps. *Gastroenterol. Res. Pract.* **2012**, *2012*, 545679. [CrossRef]
16. Cicchi, R.; Sturiale, A.; Nesi, G.; Kapsokalyvas, D.; Alemanno, G.; Tonelli, F.; Pavone, F.S. Multiphoton morpho-functional imaging of healthy colon mucosa, adenomatous polyp and adenocarcinoma. *Biomed. Opt. Express* **2013**, *4*, 1204–1213. [CrossRef]
17. He, K.; Zhao, L.; Chen, Y.; Huang, X.; Ding, Y.; Hua, H.; Liu, L.; Wang, X.; Wang, M.; Zhang, Y.; et al. Label-free multiphoton microscopic imaging as a novel real-time approach for discriminating colorectal lesions: A preliminary study. *J. Gastroenterol. Hepatol.* **2019**, *34*, 2144–2151. [CrossRef] [PubMed]
18. Pfau, P.R.; Sivak, M.V.; Chak, A.; Kinnard, M.; Wong, R.C.K.; Isenberg, G.A.; Izatt, J.A.; Rollins, A.; Westphal, V. Criteria for the diagnosis of dysplasia by endoscopic optical coherence tomography. *Gastrointest. Endosc.* **2003**, *58*, 196–202. [CrossRef] [PubMed]
19. Zagaynova, E.; Gladkova, N.; Shakhova, N.; Gelikonov, G.; Gelikonov, V. Endoscopic OCT with forward-looking probe: Clinical studies in urology and gastroenterology | Natalia Shakhova-Academia.edu. *J. Biophotonics* **2008**, *1*, 114–128. [CrossRef]
20. Iftimia, N.; Iyer, A.K.; Hammer, D.X.; Lue, N.; Mujat, M.; Pitman, M.; Ferguson, R.D.; Amiji, M. Fluorescence-guided optical coherence tomography imaging for colon cancer screening: A preliminary mouse study. *Biomed. Opt. Express* **2012**, *3*, 178–191. [CrossRef]
21. Ding, Q.; Deng, Y.; Yu, X.; Yuan, J.; Zeng, Z.; Mu, G.; Wan, X.; Zhang, J.; Zhou, W.; Huang, L.; et al. Rapid, high-resolution, label free, and 3-dimensional imaging to differentiate colorectal adenomas and non-neoplastic polyps with micro-optical coherence tomography. *Clin. Transl. Gastroenterol.* **2019**, *10*, e00049. [CrossRef]
22. Kudo, S.E.; Tamura, S.; Nakajima, T.; Yamano, H.O.; Kusaka, H.; Watanabe, H. Diagnosis of colorectal tumorous lesions by magnifying endoscopy. *Gastrointest. Endosc.* **1996**, *44*, 8–14. [CrossRef]
23. Adler, D.C.; Zhou, C.; Tsai, T.-H.; Schmitt, J.; Huang, Q.; Mashimo, H.; Fujimoto, J.G. Three-dimensional endomicroscopy of the human colon using optical coherence tomography. *Opt. Express* **2009**, *17*, 784–796. [CrossRef] [PubMed]
24. Ahsen, O.O.; Lee, H.C.; Liang, K.; Wang, Z.; Figueiredo, M.; Huang, Q.; Potsaid, B.; Jayaraman, V.; Fujimoto, J.G.; Mashimo, H. Ultrahigh-speed endoscopic optical coherence tomography and angiography enables delineation of lateral margins of endoscopic mucosal resection: A case report. *Therap. Adv. Gastroenterol.* **2017**, *10*, 931–936. [CrossRef] [PubMed]
25. Liang, K.; Ahsen, O.O.; Wang, Z.; Lee, H.-C.; Liang, W.; Potsaid, B.M.; Tsai, T.-H.; Giacomelli, M.G.; Jayaraman, V.; Mashimo, H.; et al. Endoscopic forward-viewing optical coherence tomography and angiography with MHz swept source. *Opt. Lett.* **2017**, *42*, 3193–3196. [CrossRef]
26. Zeng, Y.; Rao, B.; Chapman, W.C.; Nandy, S.; Rais, R.; González, I.; Chatterjee, D.; Mutch, M.; Zhu, Q. The Angular Spectrum of the Scattering Coefficient Map Reveals Subsurface Colorectal Cancer. *Sci. Rep.* **2019**, *9*, 1–11. [CrossRef]

27. Picón Ruiz, A.; Alvarez Gila, A.; Irusta, U.; Echazarra Huguet, J. Why deep learning performs better than classical machine learning engenering. *Dyn. Ing. Ind.* **2020**, *95*, 119–122.
28. Krizhevsky, A.; Sutskever, I.; Hinton, G.E. ImageNet Classification with Deep Convolutional Neural Networks. In *Advances in Neural Information Processing Systems 25*; Pereira, F., Burges, C.J.C., Bottou, L., Weinberger, K.Q., Eds.; Curran Associates, Inc.: Red Hook, NY, USA, 2012; pp. 1097–1105.
29. LeCun, Y.; Haffner, P.; Bottou, L.; Bengio, Y. Object recognition with gradient-based learning. In *Lecture Notes in Computer Science (Including Subseries Lecture Notes in Artificial Intelligence and Lecture Notes in Bioinformatics)*; Springer: Berlin/Heidelberg, Germany, 1999; Volume 1681, pp. 319–345.
30. Goodfellow, I.; Bengio, Y.; Courville, A. *Deep Learning*; The MIT Press: Cambridge, MA, USA, 2016.
31. LeCun, Y.A.; Bengio, Y.; Hinton, G.E. Deep learning. *Nature* **2015**, *521*, 436–444. [CrossRef] [PubMed]
32. Litjens, G.; Kooi, T.; Bejnordi, B.E.; Setio, A.A.A.; Ciompi, F.; Ghafoorian, M.; van der Laak, J.A.W.M.; van Ginneken, B.; Sánchez, C.I. A Survey on Deep Learning in Medical Image Analysis. *Med. Image Anal.* **2017**, *42*, 60–88. [CrossRef]
33. Esteva, A.; Kuprel, B.; Novoa, R.A.; Ko, J.; Swetter, S.M.; Blau, H.M.; Thrun, S. Dermatologist-level classification of skin cancer with deep neural networks. *Nature* **2017**, *542*, 115–118. [CrossRef] [PubMed]
34. Liu, X.; Faes, L.; Kale, A.U.; Wagner, S.K.; Fu, D.J.; Bruynseels, A.; Mahendiran, T.; Moraes, G.; Shamdas, M.; Kern, C.; et al. A comparison of deep learning performance against health-care professionals in detecting diseases from medical imaging: A systematic review and meta-analysis. *Lancet Digit. Health* **2019**, *1*, 271–297. [CrossRef]
35. Wei, J.W.; Suriawinata, A.A.; Vaickus, L.J.; Ren, B.; Liu, X.; Lisovsky, M.; Tomita, N.; Abdollahi, B.; Kim, A.S.; Snover, D.C.; et al. Evaluation of a Deep Neural Network for Automated Classification of Colorectal Polyps on Histopathologic Slides. *JAMA Netw. Open* **2020**, *3*, e203398. [CrossRef]
36. Medela, A.; Picon, A. Constellation loss: Improving the efficiency of deep metric learning loss functions for the optimal embedding of histopathological images. *J. Pathol. Inform.* **2020**, *11*, 38.
37. Terradillos, E.; Saratxaga, C.L.; Mattana, S.; Cicchi, R.; Pavone, F.S.; Andraka, N.; Glover, B.J.; Arbide, N.; Velasco, J.; Echezarraga, M.C.; et al. Analysis on the characterization of multiphoton microscopy images for malignant neoplastic colon lesion detection under deep learning methods. in press.
38. Sánchez-Peralta, L.F.; Picón, A.; Sánchez-Margallo, F.M.; Pagador, J.B. Unravelling the effect of data augmentation transformations in polyp segmentation. *Int. J. Comput. Assist. Radiol. Surg.* **2020**, *15*, 1975–1988. [CrossRef]
39. Sánchez-Peralta, L.F.; Pagador, J.B.; Picón, A.; Calderón, Á.J.; Polo, F.; Andraka, N.; Bilbao, R.; Glover, B.; Saratxaga, C.L.; Sánchez-Margallo, F.M. PICCOLO White-Light and Narrow-Band Imaging Colonoscopic Dataset: A Performance Comparative of Models and Datasets. *Appl. Sci.* **2020**, *10*, 8501. [CrossRef]
40. Sánchez-Peralta, L.F.; Bote-Curiel, L.; Picón, A.; Sánchez-Margallo, F.M.; Pagador, J.B. Deep learning to find colorectal polyps in colonoscopy: A systematic literature review. *Artif. Intell. Med.* **2020**, *108*, 101923. [CrossRef] [PubMed]
41. Picon, A.; Medela, A.; Sanchez-Peralta, L.F.; Cicchi, R.; Bilbao, R.; Alfieri, D.; Elola, A.; Glover, B.; Saratxaga, C.L. Autofluorescence image reconstruction and virtual staining for in-vivo optical biopsying. *IEEE Access* **2021**, *9*, 32081–32093. [CrossRef]
42. Yanagihara, R.T.; Lee, C.S.; Ting, D.S.W.; Lee, A.Y. Methodological challenges of deep learning in optical coherence tomography for retinal diseases: A review. *Transl. Vis. Sci. Technol.* **2020**, *9*, 11. [CrossRef] [PubMed]
43. Lu, W.; Tong, Y.; Yu, Y.; Xing, Y.; Chen, C.; Shen, Y. Deep learning-based automated classification of multi-categorical abnormalities from optical coherence tomography images. *Transl. Vis. Sci. Technol.* **2018**, *7*, 41. [CrossRef]
44. Jiang, Z.; Huang, Z.; Qiu, B.; Meng, X.; You, Y.; Liu, X.; Liu, G.; Zhou, C.; Yang, K.; Maier, A.; et al. Comparative study of deep learning models for optical coherence tomography angiography. *Biomed. Opt. Express* **2020**, *11*, 1580–1597. [CrossRef]
45. Singla, N.; Dubey, K.; Srivastava, V. Automated assessment of breast cancer margin in optical coherence tomography images via pretrained convolutional neural network. *J. Biophotonics* **2019**, *12*, e201800255. [CrossRef] [PubMed]
46. Zeng, Y.; Xu, S.; Chapman, W.C.; Li, S.; Alipour, Z.; Abdelal, H.; Chatterjee, D.; Mutch, M.; Zhu, Q. Real-time colorectal cancer diagnosis using PR-OCT with deep learning. *Theranostics* **2020**, *10*, 2587–2596. [CrossRef] [PubMed]
47. Lin, T.Y.; Goyal, P.; Girshick, R.; He, K.; Dollar, P. Focal Loss for Dense Object Detection. *IEEE Trans. Pattern Anal. Mach. Intell.* **2020**, *42*, 318–327. [CrossRef]
48. Amos-Landgraf, J.M.; Kwong, L.N.; Kendziorski, C.M.; Reichelderfer, M.; Torrealba, J.; Weichert, J.; Haag, J.D.; Chen, K.S.; Waller, J.L.; Gould, M.N.; et al. A target-selected Apc-mutant rat kindred enhances the modeling of familial human colon cancer. *Proc. Natl. Acad. Sci. USA* **2007**, *104*, 4036–4041. [CrossRef]
49. Irving, A.A.; Yoshimi, K.; Hart, M.L.; Parker, T.; Clipson, L.; Ford, M.R.; Kuramoto, T.; Dove, W.F.; Amos-Landgraf, J.M. The utility of Apc-mutant rats in modeling human colon cancer. *DMM Dis. Model. Mech.* **2014**, *7*, 1215–1225. [CrossRef]
50. Bote-Chacón, J.; Moreno-Lobato, B.; Sanchez-Margallo, F.M. Pilot study for the characterization of a murine model of hyperplastic growth in colon. In Proceedings of the 27th International Congress European Association of Endoscopic Surgery, Seville, Spain, 12–15 June 2019.
51. Bote-Chacón, J.; Ortega-Morán, J.F.; Pagador, B.; Moreno-Lobato, B.L.; Saratxaga, C.; Sánchez-Margallo, F.M. Validation of murine hyperplastic model of the colon. In Proceedings of the Abstracts of the first virtual Congres of the Spanish Society of Surgical Research. *Br. J. Surg.* **2022**. to be published.
52. Thorlabs CAL110C1-Spectral Domain OCT System. Available online: https://www.thorlabs.com/thorproduct.cfm?partnumber=CAL110C1 (accessed on 15 September 2020).

53. Gleed, R.D.; Ludders, J.W. *Recent Advances in Veterinary Anesthesia and Analgesia: Companion Animals*; International Veterinary Information Service: Ithaca, NY, USA, 2008.
54. Abreu, M.; Aguado, D.; Benito, J.; Gómez de Segura, I.A. Reduction of the sevoflurane minimum alveolar concentration induced by methadone, tramadol, butorphanol and morphine in rats. *Lab. Anim.* **2012**, *46*, 200–206. [CrossRef] [PubMed]
55. Flecknell, P. *Laboratory Animal Anaesthesia*; Elsevier: Amsterdam, The Netherlands, 1996.
56. Gabrecht, T.; Andrejevic-Blant, S.; Wagnières, G. Blue-Violet Excited Autofluorescence Spectroscopy and Imaging of Normal and Cancerous Human Bronchial Tissue after Formalin Fixation. *Photochem. Photobiol.* **2007**, *83*, 450–459. [CrossRef] [PubMed]
57. Chollet, F. Xception: Deep learning with depthwise separable convolutions. In Proceedings of the 30th IEEE Conference on Computer Vision and Pattern Recognition, CVPR 2017, Honolulu, HI, USA, 21–26 July 2016; Institute of Electrical and Electronics Engineers Inc.: New York, NY, USA, 2017; pp. 1800–1807.
58. Russakovsky, O.; Deng, J.; Su, H.; Krause, J.; Satheesh, S.; Ma, S.; Huang, Z.; Karpathy, A.; Khosla, A.; Bernstein, M.; et al. ImageNet Large Scale Visual Recognition Challenge. *Int. J. Comput. Vis.* **2015**, *115*, 211–252. [CrossRef]
59. Bäuerle, A.; van Onzenoodt, C.; Ropinski, T. Net2Vis-A Visual Grammar for Automatically Generating Publication-Tailored CNN Architecture Visualizations. *IEEE Trans. Vis. Comput. Graph.* **2019**, *1*. [CrossRef]
60. Otsu, N. A Threshold Selection Method from Gray-Level Histograms. *IEEE Trans. Syst. Man. Cybern.* **1979**, *9*, 62–66. [CrossRef]
61. Treuting, P.M.; Dintzis, S.M. Lower Gastrointestinal Tract. In *Comparative Anatomy and Histology*; Elsevier Inc.: Amsterdam, The Netherlands, 2012; pp. 177–192.
62. Kollár-Hunek, K.; Héberger, K. Method and model comparison by sum of ranking differences in cases of repeated observations (ties). *Chemom. Intell. Lab. Syst.* **2013**, *127*, 139–146. [CrossRef]

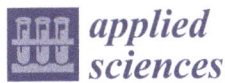

Article

Deep Learning-Based Pixel-Wise Lesion Segmentation on Oral Squamous Cell Carcinoma Images

Francesco Martino [1], Domenico D. Bloisi [2,*], Andrea Pennisi [3], Mulham Fawakherji [4], Gennaro Ilardi [1], Daniela Russo [1], Daniele Nardi [4], Stefania Staibano [1,†] and Francesco Merolla [5,†]

[1] Department of Advanced Biomedical Sciences, University of Naples Federico II, 80131 Napoli, Italy; francesco.martino@unina.it (F.M.); gennaro.ilardi@unina.it (G.I.); daniela.russo@unina.it (D.R.); stefania.staibano@unina.it (S.S.)
[2] Department of Mathematics, Computer Science, and Economics, University of Basilicata, 85100 Potenza, Italy
[3] Allianz Benelux, 1000 Brussels, Belgium; andrea.pennisi@allianz.be
[4] Department of Computer Science, Control, and Management Engineering, Sapienza University of Rome, 00185 Rome, Italy; fawakherji@diag.uniroma1.it (M.F.); nardi@diag.uniroma1.it (D.N.)
[5] Department of Medicine and Health Sciences "V. Tiberio", University of Molise, 86100 Campobasso, Italy; francesco.merolla@unimol.it
* Correspondence: domenico.bloisi@unibas.it
† Co-senior authors.

Received: 10 October 2020; Accepted: 18 November 2020; Published: 23 November 2020

Abstract: Oral squamous cell carcinoma is the most common oral cancer. In this paper, we present a performance analysis of four different deep learning-based pixel-wise methods for lesion segmentation on oral carcinoma images. Two diverse image datasets, one for training and another one for testing, are used to generate and evaluate the models used for segmenting the images, thus allowing to assess the generalization capability of the considered deep network architectures. An important contribution of this work is the creation of the Oral Cancer Annotated (ORCA) dataset, containing ground-truth data derived from the well-known Cancer Genome Atlas (TCGA) dataset.

Keywords: oral carcinoma; medical image segmentation; deep learning

---

1. Introduction

Malignant tumors of the head and neck region include a large variety of lesions, the great majority of which are squamous cell carcinomas of the oral cavity [1]. According to GLOBOCAN 2018 data on cancer [2], oral cavity malignant neoplasms, together with lip and pharynx malignancies, account for more than half-million new occurrences per year worldwide, with an estimated incidence of 5.06 cases per 100,000 inhabitants. Moreover, Oral Squamous Cell Carcinoma (OSCC) is characterized by high morbidity and mortality, and, in most countries, the survival rate after five years from the diagnosis is less than 50% of the patients [3].

The histology examination is the gold standard for the definition of these tumors. Surgical pathologists use both clinical and radiological evidence to complement their diagnoses, differentiating between benign and malignant lesions. In the last years, surgical pathology is witnessing a digital transformation thanks to (1) the increase of the processing speed of Whole Slide Images (WSI) scanners [4] and (2) the lower storage costs and better compression algorithm [5]. Consequently, WSI digital analysis is one of the most prominent and innovative topics in anatomical pathology, catching academic and industries attentions. An example of an image obtained using a WSI scanner is shown in Figure 1.

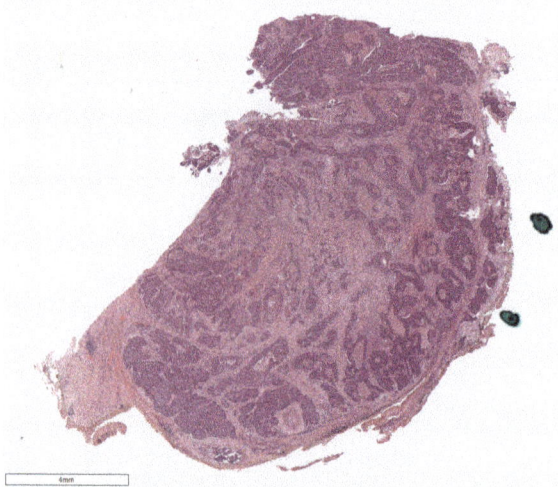

Figure 1. An example of image generated by a Whole Slide Images (WSI) scanner. The image has a dimension of 35,862 × 32,195 pixels and the file size is 213.3 MB.

However, WSI (and associated datasets) are characterized by three important limitations:

1. WSI are extremely large images, having a memory size of two gigabytes on average [6].
2. There are a few surgical pathology units that are fully digitalized and that can store a large amount of digitalized slides, although their number is increasing exponentially [7].
3. There is a small number of available image datasets and most of them are not annotated [8].

Due to the above-discussed limitations, the research activity based on Artificial Intelligence (AI) algorithms applied to WSI is still limited compared to other diagnostic imaging branches, such as radiology, but the scientific literature on the topic is growing fast and we are observing the appearance of public datasets of unannotated and annotated histopathology WSI.

In this paper, we present a performance evaluation of four different image segmentation architectures based on deep learning to obtain a pixel-wise separation between benign and malignant areas on WSI samples. In particular, we test four widely used Semantic Segmentation deep neural Networks (SSNs) on publicly available data for the detection of carcinomas. As a difference with respect to classification neural network, SSNs take as input images of arbitrary sizes and produce a correspondingly sized segmented output, without relying on local patches.

The contributions of this work are three-fold:

1. We compare four different supervised pixel-wise segmentation methods for detecting carcinoma areas in WSI using quantitative metrics. Different input formats, including separating the color channels in the RGB and Hue, Saturation, and Value (HSV) models, are taken into account in the experiments.
2. We use two different image datasets, one for training and another one for testing. This allows us to understand the real generalization capabilities of the considered SSNs.
3. We created a publicly available dataset, called Oral Cancer Annotated (ORCA) dataset, containing annotated data from the Cancer Genome Atlas (TCGA) dataset, which can be used by other researchers for testing their approaches.

The paper is organized as follows. Section 2 contains a discussion of similar approaches present in the literature. Section 3 describes the details of the proposed method, while Section 4 shows both qualitative and quantitative results obtained on publicly available data. Finally, conclusions are drawn in Section 5.

2. Related Work

Artificial intelligence (AI) algorithms have been proposed to address a wide variety of questions in medicine; e.g., for prostate Gleason score classification [9], renal cancer grading [10], breast cancer molecular subtyping [11] and their outcome prediction. Moreover, AI-based methods have been applied to the segmentation of various pathological lesions in the fields of neuropathology [12], breast cancer [13], hematopathology [14], and nephrology [15].

The above-cited studies have been conducted mainly on the most common tumors (i.e., breast or prostate), while AI-based methods have been scarcely adopted to deal with other types of cancer, despite their high incidence and mortality rates, as the Oral Squamous Cell Carcinoma (OSCC). The analysis of a recent systematic review by Mahmood et al. [16] shows that still few applications of automatic WSI analysis algorithms are available for OSCC. In particular, the survey reports 11 records about the employment of AI-based methods for the analysis of specific histological features of oral lesions: out of 11, only four papers refer to OSCCs, namely [17–20], one paper is about oral epithelial dysplasia [21], five about oral submucous fibrosis, i.e., [22–26], and one paper is about oropharyngeal squamous cell carcinoma [19]. Another recent application of machine learning algorithms on oral lesions histopathological is based on immunohistochemistry (IHC) positivity prediction [27].

Segmentation methods on WSI images have been developed mainly for nuclei segmentation [28–30], epithelium segmentation [19,24], microvessels and nerves [31], and colour-based tumour segmentation [17]. Recently, Shaban et al. [32] proposed an indirect segmentation method, through small tiles classification, with an accuracy of 95.12% (sensitivity 88.69%, specificity 97.37%).

To the best of our knowledge, there are no published results on direct OSCC segmentation using deep learning and none employing the TCGA as a source of histopathological images. This work represents a first attempt of applying well-known deep learning-based segmentation methods on the publicly available TCGA images, providing also annotations to quantitatively validate the proposed approach.

Datasets

Concerning WSI datasets, most of them have been made available for challenges, such as Camelyon [33] and HEROHE, on Kaggle or as part of larger databases. The Cancer Genome Atlas (TCGA) [34] contains publicly available data provided by the National Cancer Institute (NCI), which is the U.S. federal government's principal agency for cancer research and training, since 2006. In particular, it contains clinicopathological information and unannotated WSI of over 20,000 primary cancer covering 33 different cancer types [35].

3. Methods

Our aim is to use a supervised method to automatically segment an input WSI sample into three classes:

1. Carcinoma pixels;
2. Tissue pixels not belonging to a carcinoma;
3. Non-tissue pixels.

Figure 2 shows the functional architecture of our approach. We worked on input images having a large dimension of 4500 × 4500 pixels, which is an input dimension about ten times greater than the input dimension supported by existing segmentation SSNs. Thus, a preprocessing step is needed in order to fit the input format of the deep neural network. We tested two different pre-processing functions:

- Simple resizing, where the original input WSI sample is resized from 4500 × 4500 to 512 × 512 pixels without any other change in the color model.
- Color model change, where the WSI sample is resized to 512 × 512 pixels and the original color model is modified. For example, we tested as input for the deep neural network the use of the Red channel of the RGB model in combination with the Hue channel of the HSV model.

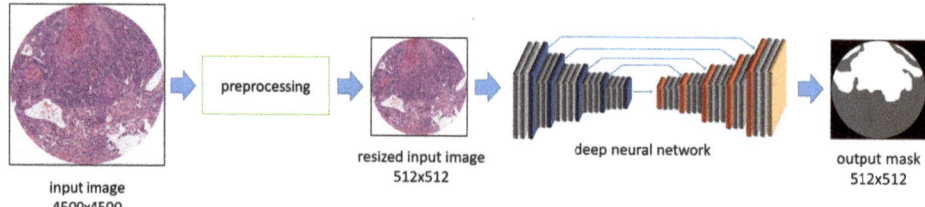

Figure 2. Functional architecture of the proposed approach.

Segmentation results obtained using the different pre-processing functions are discussed in Section 4.

3.1. Network Architectures

The core of the proposed approach consists in the use of a semantic segmentation network. We have selected four different network architectures among the most used ones:

1. SegNet [36].
2. U-Net [37].
3. U-Net with VGG16 encoder.
4. U-Net with ResNet50 encoder.

3.1.1. Segnet

SegNet is made of an encoder network and a corresponding decoder network, followed by a final pixel-wise classification layer (Figure 3). The encoder network consists of the first 13 convolutional layers of the VGG16 [38] network designed for object classification, without considering the fully connected layer in order to retain higher resolution feature maps at the deepest encoder output. In such a way, the number of parameters to train is significantly reduced. Each encoder layer has a corresponding decoder made of 13 layers. The final decoder output is fed to a multi-class soft-max classifier to produce class probabilities for each pixel independently.

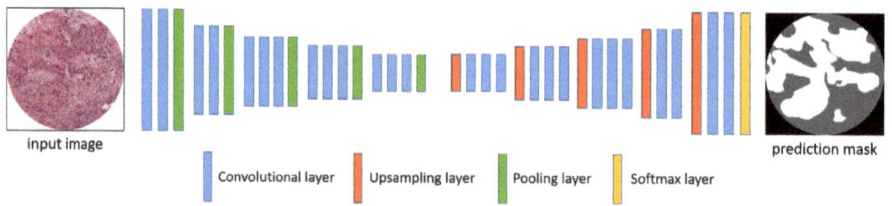

Figure 3. SegNet architecture.

3.1.2. U-Net

The architecture of the net is shown in Figure 4. The input image is downsampled to obtain a 512×512 resized image.

The encoding stage is needed to create a 512 feature vector and it is made of ten 3×3 convolutional layers, and by four 2×2 max pooling operations with stride 2. In particular, there is a repeated application of two unpadded convolutions, each followed by a rectified linear unit (ReLU) and a max pooling operation. The decoding stage (see the right side of Figure 4) is needed to obtain the predicted mask at 512×512 pixels. It is made of eight 3×3 convolutional layers and by four 2×2 transpose layers. There is a repeated application of two unpadded convolutions, each followed by a ReLU and a transpose operation. Figure 4 shows also the concatenation arcs from the encoding side to the decoding side of the network. Cropping is necessary due to the loss of border pixels in every convolution layer.

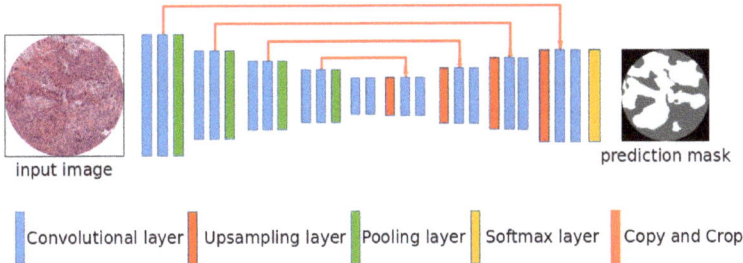

Figure 4. U-Net architecture.

3.1.3. U-Net with Different Encoders

The original U-Net consists of two paths, the first one (left side) composed of four blocks. Each block consists of a typical architecture of a convolution network, composed of repeated two 3×3 Convolutional layers followed by a rectified linear unit (ReLU) and a 2×2 max pooling layer with stride 2 as down-sampling steps. The second path (right side) represents the up-sampling path also composed of four blocks. Each block consists of an up-sampling feature map followed by concatenation with the corresponding cropped feature map from the first path followed by a double 3×3 Convolutional layer. Each convolution layer is composed of batch normalization. Between the first and the second path, there is a bottleneck block. This bottleneck is built from two convolution layers with batch normalization and dropout. In the models we applied, we replaced the first path, which is the encoder path of the network, with two different models, namely VGG16 [38] and ResNet50 [39], in order to obtain higher accuracy.

3.2. Training and Test

Two diverse datasets are used to train, validate, and test the networks. The training dataset consists of 188 annotated images of advanced OSCC derived from the digital data acquired in the Surgical Pathology Unit of the Federico II Hospital in Naples (Italy). The study was performed in agreement with Italian law. Moreover, according to the Declaration of Helsinki for studies based only on retrospective analyses on routine archival FFPE-tissue, written informed consent was acquired from the living patient at the time of surgery. The validation dataset consists of 100 annotated images from the newly created ORCA dataset (described below), while the test dataset consists of a further 100 images from the ORCA dataset also. All the images in the two datasets have been manually annotated by two of the authors of this paper that are expert pathologists (D. Russo and F. Merolla, both MD PhD and Board in Pathology) using three color labels:

1. Carcinoma pixels, colored in white.
2. Tissue pixels not belonging to a carcinoma, colored in grey.
3. Non-tissue pixels, colored in black.

The above-listed labels represent the classes learned by the deep network during the training stage. Figure 5 shows an example of annotation mask.

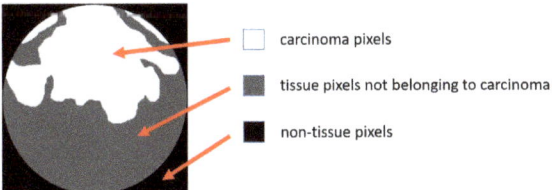

Figure 5. Example of annotation mask. Carcinoma pixels are colored in white, tissue pixels not belonging to a carcinoma are colored in grey, and non-tissue pixels are colored in black.

3.2.1. Training Data

The dataset used for training consists of a set of images collected by the Surgical Pathology Unit of the Federico II Hospital, in Naples (Italy). In particular, cases were assembled as four Tissue Micro Array and, after H&E staining, the slides were scanned with a Leica Aperio AT2 at 40× (20× optical magnification plus a 2× optical multiplier).

Slides were annotated using the Leica Aperio ImageScope software. In the first instance, to define each core, we used the ImageScope rectangle tool with a fixed size of 4500 × 4500 pixels, corresponding to nearly 1.125 mm, i.e., the size of each TMA core. Then, an expert pathologist used the pen tool to contour the tumor areas within each core. ImageScope provides an XML file as output for each WSI. RGB core images were extracted using OpenCV and OpenSlide libraries.

Concerning the annotation masks, we started by automatically detecting the tissue portion of each core using the OpenCV functions contouring and convex hull, to isolate the tissue pixels (colored in grey, as mentioned beforehand) from the background (non-tissue pixels colored in black). Then, the tumor masks (colored in white) were superimposed over the tissue pixels to draw carcinoma pixels. Finally, the masks were manually refined at pixel-size resolution.

An example of a couple <original image, annotated mask> used for the training stage is shown on the top of Figure 6.

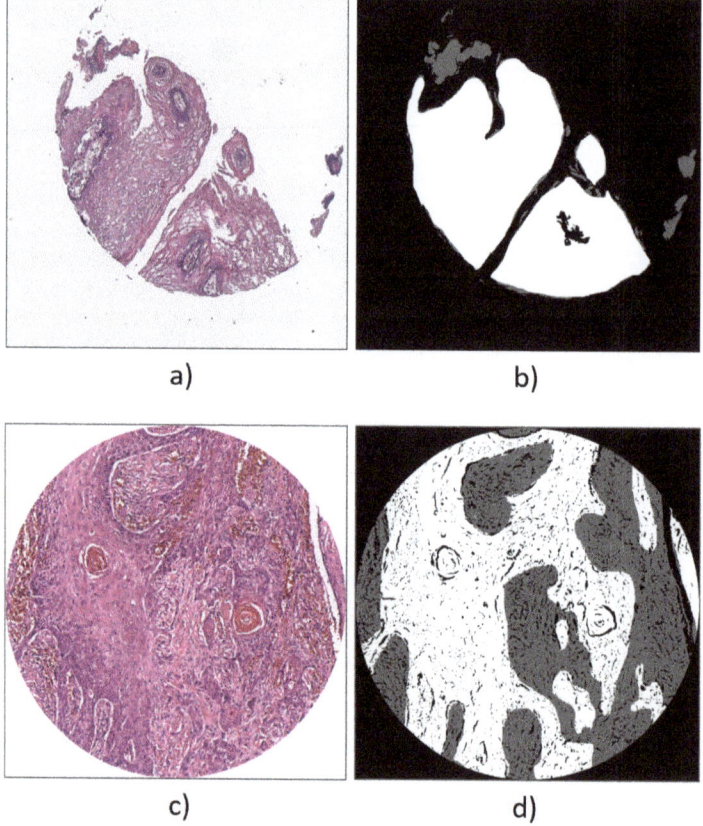

Figure 6. Top: Example of annotated data from the training dataset. (**a**) Original image. (**b**) Manually generated annotation mask. Bottom: Example of annotated data from the Oral Cancer Annotated (ORCA) dataset. (**c**) Original image. (**d**) Manually generated annotation mask.

3.2.2. ORCA Dataset

An important contribution of this work is the creation of a fully annotated dataset, called ORCA, consisting of couples of WSI samples plus corresponding annotation masks. An example of a couple <original image, annotated mask> from the ORCA dataset is shown on the bottom of Figure 6.

The original WSI samples belong to the Cancer Genome Atlas (TCGA), a landmark cancer genomics program, molecularly characterized over 20,000 primary cancer and matched normal samples spanning 33 cancer types [40]. TCGA data are publicly available for anyone in the research community to use. For each WSI included in the TCGA dataset, we defined one or two cores containing a representative tumor area. The dataset contains WSI scanned both at 20× and at 40×.

TCGA whole slide images were annotated using the Leica Aperio ImageScope software. For each image, a circular core region has been selected using the ImageScope ellipse tool, with a fixed size of 4500 × 4500 pixels in the case of the WSI scanned at 40× or 2250 × 2250 pixels in the case of WSI acquired at 20×. This allowed us to keep the same spatial dimension for all the selected cores. Then, the tumor contours have been drawn using a pen tool. The RGB images and the corresponding annotation masks were extracted using OpenCV and OpenSlide libraries.

All the couples of WSI samples plus corresponding annotation masks used in this work are available for downloading from the ORCA dataset web page at: https://sites.google.com/unibas.it/orca.

4. Experimental Results

In order to train and evaluate the networks, we split the image data into training, validation, and test sets. The training set consists of the 188 images from the Federico II Hospital plus a set of images obtained by applying a simple augmentation technique. This allows for augmenting the number of the available training samples. In particular, the data augmentation has been achieved by flipping the images vertically, horizontally, and in both ways. The final cardinality of the augmented training set is 756 images.

Each validation and test set includes 100 images from the ORCA data set. It is worth noticing that validation and test set are completely disjoint sets. In such a way, we tested the capability of the networks in generalizing the segmentation problem.

As stated above, we trained four different models:

- SegNet.
- U-Net.
- U-Net with VGG16 encoder.
- U-Net with ResNet50 encoder.

The source code of the used SegNet network is available at https://github.com/apennisi/segnet, while the source code for U-Net and its modifications is available at https://github.com/Mulham91/Deep-Learning-based-Pixel-wise-Lesion-Segmentationon-Oral-Squamous-Cell-Carcinoma-Images.

The four networks have been trained by using the Adam optimizer, with a learning rate of $1e-4$, without adopting any decay technique. The input image size has been set to 512 × 512 pixels.

For computing the loss, we used the Cross-Entropy function [41], which is a loss function widely used in deep learning. Cross entropy helps in speeding up the training for neural networks in comparison to the other losses [42]. The cross entropy for multi-class error computation is defined as follows:

$$s = -\sum_{c=1}^{M} y_{o,c} \log(p_{o,c}), \quad (1)$$

where c is the class id, o is the observation id, and p is the probability. Such a definition may also be called categorical cross entropy.

The training has been manually stopped after 60 epochs for all the considered network architectures because we noticed a trend of all the network in overfitting the training set.

We performed three kinds of experiments:

1. Using RGB images as input;
2. Taking into account the HSV color representation and concatenating the Hue channel with the Red channel from the RGB space;
3. Using the Red and Value channels.

An example of the different color models mentioned above is shown in Figure 7. The original RGB image is decomposed into single channels using the RGB and HSV color models. Then, some channels have been selected as input for the deep network. In particular, we used H + R and R + V.

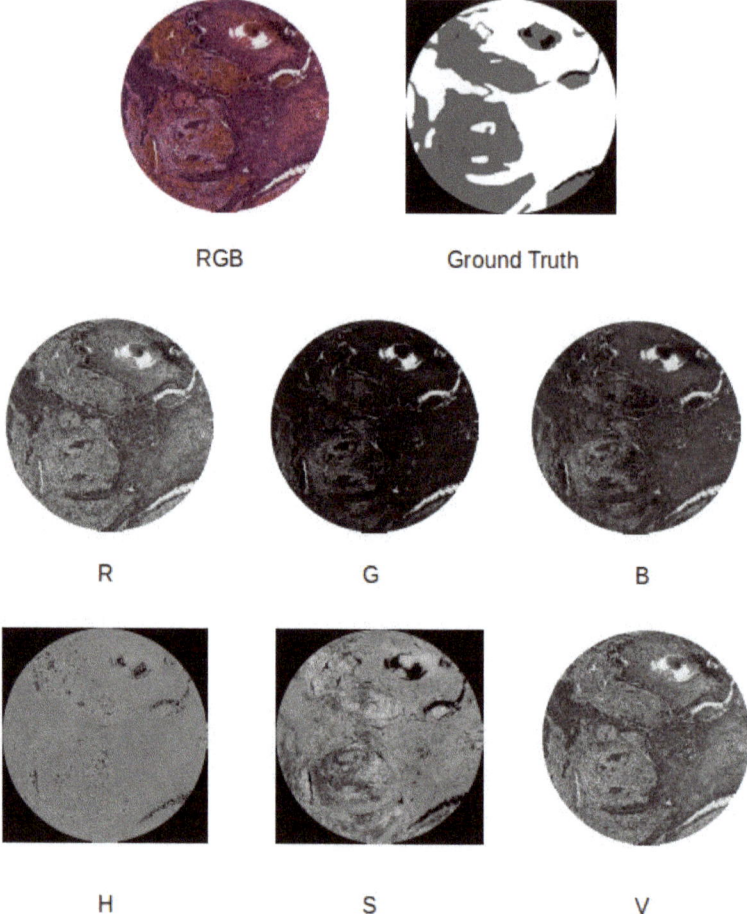

Figure 7. An example of the input images used for training the networks. First row: Original input and corresponding annotated mask. Second row: Red, Green, and Blue channels from the original RGB image. Third row: Hue, Saturation, and Value channels from the transformation of the original RGB image into Hue, Saturation, and Value (HSV).

The idea of using a multi-spectral input derives from the application of deep learning techniques in the area of precision farming, where multi-spectral inputs have denoted good performance on SSNs for the segmentation of crop and weed plants in images acquired from farming robots [43].

The prediction masks produced by the deep networks have been compared with the ground-truth annotation masks in order to measure the capability of our pipeline in generating accurate results. In particular, we have used the number of false-positive (FP), false-negative (FN), and true-positive (TP) carcinoma pixel detections as an indicator for the evaluation of the results. Figure 8 shows an example of how we computed FP, FN, and TP pixels to evaluate the predicted mask.

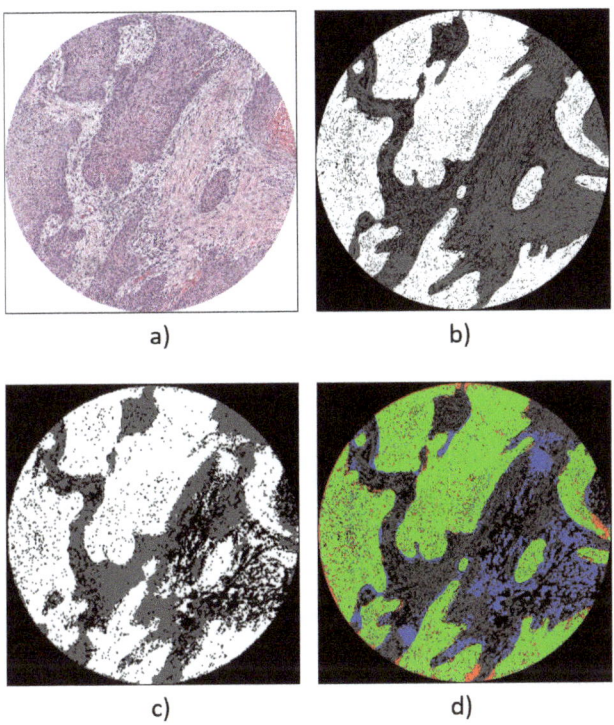

Figure 8. An example of error analysis for a test image. (**a**) The original image included in the test set. (**b**) The corresponding annotation mask, where carcinoma pixels are coloured in white. (**c**) The predicted mask generated from U-Net with ResNet50 encoder. (**d**) The coloured error mask, where green pixels are true-positive (TP) carcinoma pixels, blue are false-positives (FPs), and red are false-negatives (FNs).

4.1. Qualitative Evaluation

We evaluated the output of the trained network, in the first instance, by visual inspection. This allowed us to interpret the results and judge them in the light of the pathologist's experience and diagnostic reasoning in histopathology.

In most cases, we observed that the areas reported as false positives (blue pixels in Figure 8d) actually corresponded to small nests of stromal infiltration, located in correspondence with the tumor invasion front.

Vice versa, we observed that a portion of the pixels reported as false negatives actually referred to small areas of stroma within the tumor area. For example, by observing the colored mask in Figure 8d, it is visible that the stromal area within the tumor is considered as a set of false-negative pixels (coloured in red) even if they should be considered as true positives.

Given the discussion above, from a qualitative point of view, the algorithm has often reported pixels relating to areas of intense inflammatory infiltrate as false positives. However, single interspersed lymphocytes in the peritumor stroma were not per se a problem in the interpretation of the image.

Tumor grading was another determining factor in the efficiency of the algorithm. In fact, the trained network recognized with difficulty the highly differentiated tumor areas, with a prevalence of keratin pearls. This last factor could be attributable to the fact that the dataset used for the training was mainly composed of a series of high grade advanced squamous carcinomas.

4.2. Quantitative Results

To obtain a quantitative measure of the segmentation performance achieved by the four deep networks, we used the Mean Intersection-Over-Union (mIOU) metric. MIOU is one of the most common metrics for evaluating semantic image segmentation tasks. In particular, we first computed the IOU for each semantic class, namely carcinoma, tissue non-carcinoma, and non-tissue, and then computed the average over all classes. The $mIOU$ is defined as follows:

$$mIOU = \frac{1}{C} \sum_{i=1}^{C} \frac{TP_j}{TP_j + FP_j + FN_j},$$
(2)

where TP is true-positive, FP is false-positive, FN is false-negative, and C is the total number of classes.

Table 1 shows the quantitative results of the semantic segmentation on three different inputs: RGB, (Red + Hue), and (Red + Value). The results show that the use of the combination (Red + Value) generates better results than (Red + Hue) input. Moreover, a deeper network, such as U-Net modified with ResNet50 as encoder, performs better than the original U-Net (having a more shallow encoder).

Table 1. Pixel-wise segmentation results.

Training Input	SSN Type	MIoU	IOU Non-Tissue	Tissue Non-Carcinoma	Carcinoma
RGB	SegNet	0.51	0.74	0.49	0.30
	U-Net	0.58	0.79	0.52	0.45
	U-Net + VGG16	0.64	0.84	0.56	0.45
	U-Net + ResNet50	0.67	0.85	0.59	0.56
Red + Hue	SegNet	0.49	0.70	0.48	0.30
	U-Net	0.55	0.78	0.50	0.38
	U-Net + VGG16	0.33	0.22	0.28	0.53
	U-Net + ResNet50	0.57	0.80	0.48	0.43
Red + Value	SegNet	0.54	0.72	0.49	0.40
	U-Net	0.57	0.78	0.49	0.46
	U-Net + VGG16	0.62	0.79	0.50	0.55
	U-Net + ResNet50	0.63	0.80	0.52	0.56

4.3. Discussion

The histological evaluation of Hematoxylin Eosin stained slides from tumor samples, carried out by an experienced pathologist on an optical microscope, is a mandatory step in the diagnostic, prognostic and therapeutic pathway of patients suffering from squamous cell carcinoma of the oral cavity. To date, for the histological diagnosis of OSCCs, the gold standard is the visual analysis of histological preparations, stained with hematoxylin and eosin; tumor recognition basically takes place on the basis of the qualitative assessment of architectural characteristics of the neoplastic tissue, based on the wealth of knowledge pathologist's own. The qualitative assessment is subjective and can suffer from inter-individual variability, especially in borderline situations that are difficult to interpret. The use of a segmentation algorithm could minimize the interpretative variability and speed up the pathologists' work, providing they with a screening tool, particularly useful in those cases in which the histopathological diagnosis must be carried out on the extensive sampling of complex surgical samples that involve the generation of multiple blocks of formalin-fixed and paraffin-embedded tissue samples, from which numerous slides stained with hematoxylin and eosin are obtained.

Based on the presented results, our contribution is composed of: (i) a novel dataset, the ORCA set, which will allow us to conduct new studies on Oral Squamous Cell Carcinoma. Particularly, the dataset is composed of annotation from the TCGA dataset, a full comprehensive dataset enriched, as well as with diagnostic slide, with clinicopathological information and molecular biology data. This could facilitate the development of molecular characterization deep learning algorithms; (ii) our method relies on 2250×2250 and 4500×4500 images, without a tiling processing. Even though an improvement in its accuracy is mandatory for clinical practice, the utilization of so large images can hugely reduce time-demand for a WSI, making our approach easily scalable to clinical routine, when hundreds of slides need to be processed each day; (iii) after demanded improvements and a clinical trial, this kind of algorithm may be part of clinical practice via L.I.S. integration, fastening OSCC diagnosis and helping pathologists to identify OSCC areas on WSI. Indeed, we foresee to extend our method on lymphonodal metastasis, giving the pathologist an easy way to detect small tumor islands, and on distant metastasis, supporting the pathologist with cases of suspect metastasis of OSCC primary tumor.

We intend to propose this artificial intelligence algorithm as a Computer-Aided Diagnostic, aware that it cannot replace the pathologist in his routine activity, but that it will be able to provide they with valid help, especially for those who find themselves working in generalist diagnostic centres on the territory, not specialized in the diagnosis of an infrequent but extremely lethal disease.

5. Conclusions

In this work, we created a dataset called ORCA, containing annotated data from the TCGA dataset, to compare four different deep learning-based architectures for oral cancer segmentation, namely: SegNet, U-Net, U-Net with VGG16 encoder, and U-Net with ResNet50 encoder. The peculiarity of this work consists of the use of a training set completely different from the test data. In such a way, we tested the capability of the networks in generalizing the problem, providing promising segmentation results.

Despite the non-optimal results, to the best of our knowledge, this is the first attempt to use an automatic segmentation algorithm for oral squamous cell carcinoma and it represents an important novelty to this pathology. Furthermore, the publically-available ORCA dataset will facilitate the development of new algorithms and will boost the research on computational approaches to OSCC.

As future directions, we will aim at enlarging the training set and at making it publicly available. In this work, we considered color transformation by using a combination of HSV and RGB color models as a method for creating a multi-channel input. This was done because the group of pathologists that are authors of this work noticed that HSV color space contains a lot of visually distinguishing features about tumor cells. We did not use color modifications for augmenting the data. However, this is an interesting aspect that will be investigated in future work. Moreover, we foresee to improve our model to achieve a result that may be transferred to clinical practice.

Author Contributions: D.D.B., A.P. and F.M. (Francesco Merolla) conceived and designed the experiments; M.F. and F.M. (Francesco Martino) performed the experiments; F.M. (Francesco Merolla) and D.R. analyzed the data; G.I. contributed reagents/materials/analysis tools; S.S. and D.N. provide a critical review of the paper. All authors have read and agreed to the published version of the manuscript.

Funding: Our research has been supported by a POR Campania FESR 2014-2020 grant; "Technological Platform: eMORFORAD-Campania" grant PG/2017/0623667.

Acknowledgments: We thank Valerio Pellegrini for his contribution in the annotation of the dataset images.

Conflicts of Interest: The authors declare no conflict of interest.

References

1. Ettinger, K.S.; Ganry, L.; Fernandes, R.P. Oral Cavity Cancer. *Oral Maxillofac. Surg. Clin. N. Am.* **2019**, *31*, 13–29. [CrossRef]
2. The Global Cancer Observatory. Available online: https://gco.iarc.fr/ (accessed on 9 October 2020).

3. Bray, F.; Ferlay, J.; Soerjomataram, I.; Siegel, R.L.; Torre, L.A.; Jemal, A. Global cancer statistics 2018: GLOBOCAN estimates of incidence and mortality worldwide for 36 cancers in 185 countries. *CA Cancer J. Clin.* **2018**, *68*, 394–424. [CrossRef] [PubMed]
4. Pantanowitz, L.; Evans, A.; Pfeifer, J.; Collins, L.; Valenstein, P.; Kaplan, K.; Wilbur, D.; Colgan, T. Review of the current state of whole slide imaging in pathology. *J. Pathol. Inform.* **2011**, *2*, 36. [CrossRef] [PubMed]
5. Helin, H.; Tolonen, T.; Ylinen, O.; Tolonen, P.; Näpänkangas, J.; Isola, J. Optimized JPEG 2000 compression for efficient storage of histopathological whole-Slide images. *J. Pathol. Inform.* **2018**, *9*. [CrossRef]
6. Hanna, M.G.; Reuter, V.E.; Hameed, M.R.; Tan, L.K.; Chiang, S.; Sigel, C.; Hollmann, T.; Giri, D.; Samboy, J.; Moradel, C.; et al. Whole slide imaging equivalency and efficiency study: Experience at a large academic center. *Mod. Pathol.* **2019**, *32*, 916–928. [CrossRef]
7. Griffin, J.; Treanor, D. Digital pathology in clinical use: Where are we now and what is holding us back? *Histopathology* **2017**, *70*, 134–145. [CrossRef]
8. Dimitriou, N.; Arandjelović, O.; Caie, P.D. Deep Learning for Whole Slide Image Analysis: An Overview. *Front. Med.* **2019**, *6*, 264. [CrossRef]
9. Xu, H.; Park, S.; Hwang, T.H. Computerized Classification of Prostate Cancer Gleason Scores from Whole Slide Images. *IEEE/ACM Trans. Comput. Biol. Bioinform.* **2019**. [CrossRef]
10. Tian, K.; Rubadue, C.A.; Lin, D.I.; Veta, M.; Pyle, M.E.; Irshad, H.; Heng, Y.J. Automated clear cell renal carcinoma grade classification with prognostic significance. *PLoS ONE* **2019**, *14*. [CrossRef]
11. Jaber, M.I.; Song, B.; Taylor, C.; Vaske, C.J.; Benz, S.C.; Rabizadeh, S.; Soon-Shiong, P.; Szeto, C.W. A deep learning image-based intrinsic molecular subtype classifier of breast tumors reveals tumor heterogeneity that may affect survival. *Breast Cancer Res.* **2020**, *22*. [CrossRef]
12. Tang, Z.; Chuang, K.V.; DeCarli, C.; Jin, L.W.; Beckett, L.; Keiser, M.J.; Dugger, B.N. Interpretable classification of Alzheimer's disease pathologies with a convolutional neural network pipeline. *Nat. Commun.* **2019**, *10*. [CrossRef]
13. Guo, Z.; Liu, H.; Ni, H.; Wang, X.; Su, M.; Guo, W.; Wang, K.; Jiang, T.; Qian, Y. A Fast and Refined Cancer Regions Segmentation Framework in Whole-slide Breast Pathological Images. *Sci. Rep.* **2019**, *9*. [CrossRef]
14. Nielsen, F.S.; Pedersen, M.J.; Olsen, M.V.; Larsen, M.S.; Røge, R.; Jørgensen, A.S. Automatic Bone Marrow Cellularity Estimation in H&E Stained Whole Slide Images. *Cytom. Part A* **2019**, *95*, 1066–1074. [CrossRef]
15. Bueno, G.; Fernandez-Carrobles, M.M.; Gonzalez-Lopez, L.; Deniz, O. Glomerulosclerosis identification in whole slide images using semantic segmentation. *Comput. Methods Programs Biomed.* **2020**, *184*. [CrossRef]
16. Mahmood, H.; Shaban, M.; Indave, B.I.; Santos-Silva, A.R.; Rajpoot, N.; Khurram, S.A. Use of artificial intelligence in diagnosis of head and neck precancerous and cancerous lesions: A systematic review. *Oral Oncol.* **2020**, *110*, 104885. [CrossRef]
17. Sun, Y.N.; Wang, Y.Y.; Chang, S.C.; Wu, L.W.; Tsai, S.T. Color-based tumor tissue segmentation for the automated estimation of oral cancer parameters. *Microsc. Res. Tech.* **2009**, *73*. [CrossRef]
18. Rahman, T.Y.; Mahanta, L.B.; Chakraborty, C.; Das, A.K.; Sarma, J.D. Textural pattern classification for oral squamous cell carcinoma. *J. Microsc.* **2018**, *269*, 85–93. [CrossRef]
19. Fouad, S.; Randell, D.; Galton, A.; Mehanna, H.; Landini, G. Unsupervised morphological segmentation of tissue compartments in histopathological images. *PLoS ONE* **2017**, *12*, e0188717. [CrossRef]
20. Das, D.K.; Bose, S.; Maiti, A.K.; Mitra, B.; Mukherjee, G.; Dutta, P.K. Automatic identification of clinically relevant regions from oral tissue histological images for oral squamous cell carcinoma diagnosis. *Tissue Cell* **2018**, *53*, 111–119. [CrossRef]
21. Baik, J.; Ye, Q.; Zhang, L.; Poh, C.; Rosin, M.; MacAulay, C.; Guillaud, M. Automated classification of oral premalignant lesions using image cytometry and Random Forests-based algorithms. *Cell. Oncol.* **2014**, *37*. [CrossRef]
22. Krishnan, M.M.R.; Venkatraghavan, V.; Acharya, U.R.; Pal, M.; Paul, R.R.; Min, L.C.; Ray, A.K.; Chatterjee, J.; Chakraborty, C. Automated oral cancer identification using histopathological images: A hybrid feature extraction paradigm. *Micron* **2012**, *43*. [CrossRef]

23. Krishnan, M.M.R.; Shah, P.; Chakraborty, C.; Ray, A.K. Statistical analysis of textural features for improved classification of oral histopathological images. *J. Med. Syst.* **2012**, *36*, 865–881. [CrossRef]
24. Krishnan, M.M.R.; Choudhary, A.; Chakraborty, C.; Ray, A.K.; Paul, R.R. Texture based segmentation of epithelial layer from oral histological images. *Micron* **2011**, *42*. [CrossRef]
25. Krishnan, M.M.R.; Pal, M.; Bomminayuni, S.K.; Chakraborty, C.; Paul, R.R.; Chatterjee, J.; Ray, A.K. Automated classification of cells in sub-epithelial connective tissue of oral sub-mucous fibrosis-An SVM based approach. *Comput. Biol. Med.* **2009**, *39*, 1096–1104. [CrossRef]
26. Mookiah, M.R.K.; Shah, P.; Chakraborty, C.; Ray, A.K. Brownian motion curve-based textural classification and its application in cancer diagnosis. *Anal. Quant. Cytol. Histol.* **2011**, *33*, 158–168.
27. Martino, F.; Varricchio, S.; Russo, D.; Merolla, F.; Ilardi, G.; Mascolo, M.; Dell'aversana, G.O.; Califano, L.; Toscano, G.; Pietro, G.D.; et al. A machine-learning approach for the assessment of the proliferative compartment of solid tumors on hematoxylin-eosin-stained sections. *Cancers* **2020**, *12*, 1344. [CrossRef]
28. Graham, S.; Vu, Q.D.; Raza, S.E.; Azam, A.; Tsang, Y.W.; Kwak, J.T.; Rajpoot, N. Hover-Net: Simultaneous segmentation and classification of nuclei in multi-tissue histology images. *Med. Image Anal.* **2019**, *58*, 101563. [CrossRef]
29. Raza, S.E.; Cheung, L.; Shaban, M.; Graham, S.; Epstein, D.; Pelengaris, S.; Khan, M.; Rajpoot, N.M. Micro-Net: A unified model for segmentation of various objects in microscopy images. *Med. Image Anal.* **2019**, *52*, 160–173. [CrossRef]
30. Rahman, T.Y.; Mahanta, L.B.; Das, A.K.; Sarma, J.D. Automated oral squamous cell carcinoma identification using shape, texture and color features of whole image strips. *Tissue Cell* **2020**, *63*. [CrossRef]
31. Fraz, M.M.; Khurram, S.A.; Graham, S.; Shaban, M.; Hassan, M.; Loya, A.; Rajpoot, N.M. FABnet: Feature attention-based network for simultaneous segmentation of microvessels and nerves in routine histology images of oral cancer. *Neural Comput. Appl.* **2020**, *32*, 9915–9928. [CrossRef]
32. Shaban, M.; Khurram, S.A.; Fraz, M.M.; Alsubaie, N.; Masood, I.; Mushtaq, S.; Hassan, M.; Loya, A.; Rajpoot, N.M. A Novel Digital Score for Abundance of Tumour Infiltrating Lymphocytes Predicts Disease Free Survival in Oral Squamous Cell Carcinoma. *Sci. Rep.* **2019**, *9*, 1–13. [CrossRef]
33. Litjens, G.; Bandi, P.; Bejnordi, B.E.; Geessink, O.; Balkenhol, M.; Bult, P.; Halilovic, A.; Hermsen, M.; van de Loo, R.; Vogels, R.; et al. 1399 H&E-stained sentinel lymph node sections of breast cancer patients: The CAMELYON dataset. *GigaScience* **2018**, *7*, 1–8. [CrossRef]
34. The Cancer Genome Atlas (TCGA). Available online: https://www.cancer.gov/about-nci/organization/ccg/research/structural-genomics/tcga (accessed on 9 October 2020).
35. Weinstein, J.N.; The Cancer Genome Atlas Research Network; Collisson, E.A.; Mills, G.B.; Shaw, K.R.; Ozenberger, B.A.; Ellrott, K.; Shmulevich, I.; Sander, C.; Stuart, J.M. The cancer genome atlas pan-cancer analysis project. *Nat. Genet.* **2013**, *45*, 1113–1120. [CrossRef] [PubMed]
36. Badrinarayanan, V.; Kendall, A.; Cipolla, R. SegNet: A Deep Convolutional Encoder-Decoder Architecture for Image Segmentation. *IEEE Trans. Pattern Anal. Mach. Intell.* **2017**, *39*, 2481–2495.
37. Ronneberger, O.; Fischer, P.; Brox, T. U-Net: Convolutional Networks for Biomedical Image Segmentation. In Proceedings of the International Conference on Medical Image Computing and Computer-Assisted Intervention, Munich, Germany, 5–9 October 2015; pp. 234–241.
38. Simonyan, K.; Zisserman, A. Very Deep Convolutional Networks for Large Scale Image Recognition. In Proceedings of the International Conference on Learning Representations, San Diego, CA, USA, 7–9 May 2015.
39. He, K.; Zhang, X.; Ren, S.; Sun, J. Deep Residual Learning for Image Recognition. In Proceedings of the IEEE Conference on Computer Vision and Pattern Recognition (CVPR), Las Vegas, NV, USA, 27–30 June 2016.
40. The National Cancer Institute (NCI). Available online: https://www.cancer.gov/ (accessed on 25 September 2020).
41. Janocha, K.; Czarnecki, W.M. On Loss Functions for Deep Neural Networks in Classification. *arXiv* **2017**, arXiv:1702.05659.

42. Sainath, T.N.; Kingsbury, B.; Soltau, H.; Ramabhadran, B. Optimization Techniques to Improve Training Speed of Deep Neural Networks for Large Speech Tasks. *IEEE Trans. Audio Speech Lang. Process.* **2013**, *21*, 2267–2276.
43. Fawakherji, M.; Potena, C.; Pretto, A.; Bloisi, D.D.; Nardi, D. Multi-Spectral Image Synthesis for Crop/Weed Segmentation in Precision Farming. *arXiv* **2020**, arXiv:2009.05750.

Publisher's Note: MDPI stays neutral with regard to jurisdictional claims in published maps and institutional affiliations.

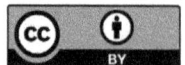

© 2020 by the authors. Licensee MDPI, Basel, Switzerland. This article is an open access article distributed under the terms and conditions of the Creative Commons Attribution (CC BY) license (http://creativecommons.org/licenses/by/4.0/).

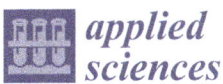

Article

An Efficient Lightweight CNN and Ensemble Machine Learning Classification of Prostate Tissue Using Multilevel Feature Analysis

Subrata Bhattacharjee [1], Cho-Hee Kim [2], Deekshitha Prakash [1], Hyeon-Gyun Park [1], Nam-Hoon Cho [3] and Heung-Kook Choi [1,*]

1. Department of Computer Engineering, u-AHRC, Inje University, Gimhae 50834, Korea; subrata_bhattacharjee@outlook.com (S.B.); deeskhithadp96@gmail.com (D.P.); gusrbs82@gmail.com (H.-G.P.)
2. Department of Digital Anti-Aging Healthcare, Inje University, Gimhae 50834, Korea; chgmlrla0917@naver.com
3. Department of Pathology, Yonsei University Hospital, Seoul 03722, Korea; cho1988@yumc.yonsei.ac.kr
* Correspondence: cschk@inje.ac.kr; Tel.: +82-10-6733-3437

Received: 23 September 2020; Accepted: 10 November 2020; Published: 12 November 2020

Abstract: Prostate carcinoma is caused when cells and glands in the prostate change their shape and size from normal to abnormal. Typically, the pathologist's goal is to classify the staining slides and differentiate normal from abnormal tissue. In the present study, we used a computational approach to classify images and features of benign and malignant tissues using artificial intelligence (AI) techniques. Here, we introduce two lightweight convolutional neural network (CNN) architectures and an ensemble machine learning (EML) method for image and feature classification, respectively. Moreover, the classification using pre-trained models and handcrafted features was carried out for comparative analysis. The binary classification was performed to classify between the two grade groups (benign vs. malignant) and quantile-quantile plots were used to show their predicted outcomes. Our proposed models for deep learning (DL) and machine learning (ML) classification achieved promising accuracies of 94.0% and 92.0%, respectively, based on non-handcrafted features extracted from CNN layers. Therefore, these models were able to predict nearly perfectly accurately using few trainable parameters or CNN layers, highlighting the importance of DL and ML techniques and suggesting that the computational analysis of microscopic anatomy will be essential to the future practice of pathology.

Keywords: prostate carcinoma; microscopic; convolutional neural network; machine learning; deep learning; handcrafted

1. Introduction

Image classification and analysis has become popular in recent years, especially for medical images. Cancer diagnosis and grading are often performed and evaluated using AI as these processes have become increasingly complex, because of growth in cancer incidence and the numbers of specific treatments. The analysis and classification of prostate cancer (PCa) are among the most challenging and difficult. PCa is the second most commonly diagnosed cancer among men in the USA and Europe, affecting approximately 25% of patients with cancer in the Western world [1]. PCa is a type of cancer that has always been an important challenge for pathologists and medical practitioners, with respect to detection, analysis, diagnosis, and treatment. Recently, researchers have analyzed PCa in young Korean men (<50 years of age), considering the pathological features of radical prostatectomy specimens and biochemical recurrence of PCa [2].

In the United States, thousands of people exhibit PCa. In 2017, there were approximately 161,360 new cases and 26,730 deaths, constituting 19% of all new cancer cases and 8% of all cancer deaths [3]. Therefore, it is important to detect PCa at an early stage to increase the survival rate. Currently, for the clinical diagnosis of PCa, methods that are performed in hospitals include a prostate-specific antigen test, digital rectal exam, trans-rectal ultrasound, and magnetic resonance imaging. Core needle biopsy examination is a common and useful technique, performed by insertion of a thin, hollow needle into the prostate gland to remove a tissue sample [4–6]. However, PCa diagnosis via microscopic biopsy images is challenging. Therefore, diagnostic accuracy may vary among pathologists.

Generally, in histopathology sections, pathologists categorize stained microscopy biopsy images into benign and malignant. To carry out PCa grading, pathologists use the Gleason grading system, which was originally based on the sum of the two Gleason scores for the most common so-called Gleason patterns (GPs). Many studies conclude that this is the recommended methodology for grading PCa [7]. The Gleason grading system defines five histological patterns from GP 1 (well differentiated) to GP 5 (poorly differentiated), with a focus on the shapes of atypical glands [8–11]. During the grossing study, the tumor affected in the prostate gland is extracted by the pathologist for examination under a microscope for cancerous cells [12,13]. In this cell culturing process, the tissues are stained with hematoxylin and eosin (H&E) compounds, yielding a combination of dark blue and bright pink colors, respectively [14–18]. In digital pathology, there are some protocols that every pathologist follows for preparing and staining the tissue slides. However, the acquisition systems and staining process vary from one pathologist to another. The generated tissue images with the variations in colour intensity and artifacts could impact the classification accuracy of the analysis [19,20].

DL and ML in AI have recently shown excellent performance in the classification of medical images. These techniques are used for computer vision tasks (e.g., segmentation, object detection, and image classification) and pattern recognition exploiting handcrafted features from a large-scale database, thus allowing new predictions from existing data [21–24]. DL is a class of ML algorithms, where multiple layers are used to extract higher-level features gradually from the raw input. ML is a branch of AI concentrated on application building that learns from data. ML algorithms are trained to learn features and patterns in huge amounts of data to make predictions based on new data. Both DL and ML have shown promising results in the field of medical imaging and have the potential to assist pathologists and radiologists with an accurate diagnosis; this may save time and minimize the costs of diagnosis [25–28]. For image classification, DL models are built to train, validate, and test thousands of images of different types for accurate prediction. These models consist of many layers through which a CNN transforms the images using functions such as convolution, kernel initialization, pooling, activation, padding, batch normalization, and stride.

The combination of image-feature engineering and ML classification has shown remarkable performance in terms of medical image analysis and classification. In contrast, CNN adaptively learns various image features to perform image transformation, focusing on features that are highly predictive for a specific learning objective. For instance, images of benign and malignant tissues could be presented to a network composed of convolutional layers with different numbers of filters that detect computational features and highlight the pixel pattern in each image. Based on these patterns, the network could use sigmoid and softmax classifiers to learn the extracted and important features, respectively. In DL, the "pipeline" of CNN's processing (i.e., from inputs to any output prediction) is opaque, performed automatically like a passage through a "black box" tunnel, where the user remains fully unaware of the process details. It is difficult to examine a CNN layer-by-layer. Therefore, each layer's visualization results and prediction mechanism are challenging to interpret.

The present paper proposes a pipeline for tissue image classification using DL and ML techniques. We developed two lightweight CNN (LWCNN) models for automatic detection of the GP in histological sections of PCa and extracted the non-handcrafted texture features from the CNN layers to classify these using an ensemble ML (EML) method. Color pre-processing was performed for enhancing images. To carry out a comparative analysis, the two types of hand-designed [29] features, such as the opposite color local binary patterns (OCLBP) [30] and improved OCLBP (IOCLBP) [30] were extracted and pre-trained models (VGG-16, ResNet-50, Inception-V3, and DenseNet-121) [31] were used for EML and DL classification, respectively. To avoid the complexity and build lightweight DL models, we used a few hidden layers and trainable parameters, and therefore, the models were named LWCNN.

The DL models were trained several times on the same histopathology dataset using different parameters and filters. For each round of training, we fine-tuned the hyperparameters, optimization function, and activation function to improve the model performance, including its accuracy. Binary classification is critical for PCa diagnosis because the goal of the pathologist is to identify whether each tumor is benign or malignant [32]. We generated a class activation map (CAM) using predicted images and created a heat map to visualize the method by which the LWCNN learned to recognize the pixel pattern (image texture) based on activation functions, thus interpreting the decision of the neural network. The CAM visualization results of the training and testing were difficult to interpret because CNNs are black-box models [33,34].

2. Related Work

A CNN was first used on medical images by Lo et al. [35,36]. Their model (LeNet) succeeded in a real-world application and could recognize hand-written digits [37]. Subsequent CNN-based methods showed the potential for automated image classification and prediction, especially after the introduction of AlexNet, a system that won the ImageNet challenge. In this era, the categorizing and auto-detection of cancer in the histological sections using machine assistance have shown excellent performance in the field of early detection of cancer.

Zheng et al. [38] developed a new CNN-based architecture for histopathological images, using the 3D multiparametric MRI data provided by PROSTATEx challenge. Data augmentation was performed through 3D rotation and slicing, to incorporate the 3D information of the lesion. They achieved the second-highest AUC (0.84) in the PROSTATEx challenge, which shows the great potential of deep learning for cancer imaging.

Han et al. [39] used breast cancer samples from the BreaKHis dataset to perform multi-classification using subordinate classes of breast cancer (ductal carcinoma, fibroadenoma, lobular carcinoma, adenosis, Phyllodes tumor, tubular adenoma, mucinous carcinoma, and papillary carcinoma). The author developed a new deep learning model and has achieved remarkable performance with an average accuracy of 93.2% on a large-scale dataset.

Kumar et al. [12] performed k-means segmentation to separate the background cells from the microscopy biopsy images. They extracted morphological and textural features from for automated detection and classification of cancer. They used different types of machine learning classifiers (random forest, Support vector machine, fuzzy k-nearest neighbor, and k-nearest neighbor) to classify connectivity, epithelial, muscular, and nervous tissues. Finally, the author obtained an average accuracy of 92.19% based on their proposed approach using a k-nearest neighbor classifier.

Abraham et al. [40] used multiparametric magnetic resonance images and presented a novel method for the grading of prostate cancer. They used VGG-16 CNN and an ordinal class classifier with J48 as the base classifier. The author used the PROSTATAx-2 2017 grand challenge dataset for their research work. Their method achieved a positive predictive value of 90.8%.

Yoo et al. [3] proposed an automated CNN-based pipeline for prostate cancer detection using diffusion-weighted magnetic resonance imaging (DWI) for each patient. They used a total of 427 patients as the dataset, out of these, 175 with PCa and 252 patients without PCa. The author used five CNNs based on the ResNet architecture and extracted first order statical features for classification. The analysis was carried out based on a slice- and patient-level. Finally, their proposed pipeline achieved the best result (AUC of 87%) using CNN1.

Turki [41] performed machine learning classification for cancer detection and used a data sample of colon, liver, thyroid cancer. They applied different ML algorithms, such as deep boost, AdaBoost, XgBoost, and support vector machines. The performance of the algorithms was evaluated using the area under the curve (AUC) and accuracy on real clinical data used classification.

Veta et al. [42] proposed different methods for the analysis of breast cancer histopathology images. They discussed different techniques for tissue image analysis and processing like tissue components segmentation, nuclei detection, tubules segmentation, mitotic detection, and computer-aided diagnosis. Before discussing the different image analysis algorithms, the author gave an overview of the tissue preparation, slide staining processes, and digitization of histological slides. In this paper, their approach is to perform clustering or supervised classification to acquire binary or probability maps for the different stains.

Moradi et al. [43] performed prostate cancer detection based on different image analysis techniques. The author used ultrasound, MRI, and histopathology images, and among these, ultrasound images were selected for cancer detection. For the classification of prostate cancer, feature extraction was carried out using the ultrasound echo radio-frequency (RF) signals, B-scan images, and Doppler images.

Alom et al. [44] proposed a deep CNN (DCNN) model for breast cancer classification. The model was developed based on the three powerful CNN architecture by combining the strength of the inception network (Inception-v4), the residual network (ResNet), and the recurrent convolutional neural network (RCNN). Thus, their proposed model was named as inception recurrent residual convolution neural network (IRRCNN). They used two publicly available datasets including BreakHis and Breast Cancer (BC) classification challenge 2015. The test results were compared against the existing state-of-art models for image-based, patch-based, image-level, and patient-level classification.

Wang et al. [45] proposed a novel method for the classification of colorectal cancer histopathological images. The author developed a novel bilinear convolutional neural network (BCNN) model that consists of two CNNs, and the outputs of the CNN layers are multiplied with the outer product at each spatial domain. Color deconvolution was performed to separate the tissue components (hematoxylin and eosin) for BCNN classification. Their proposed model performed better than the traditional CNN by classifying colorectal cancer images into eight different classes.

Bianconi et al. [20] compared the combination effect of six different colour pre-processing methods and 12 colour texture features on the patch-based classification of H&E stained images. They found that classification performance was poor using the generated colour descriptors. However, they achieved promising results using some pre-processing methods such as co-occurrence matrices, Gabor filters, and Local Binary Patterns.

Kather et al. [31] investigated the usefulness of image texture features, pre-trained convolutional networks against variants of local binary patterns for classifying different types of tissue sub-regions, namely stroma, epithelium, necrosis, and lymphocytes. They used seven different datasets of histological images for classifying the handcrafted and non-handcrafted features using standard classifiers (e.g., support vector machines) to obtain overall accuracy between 95% and 99%.

3. Tissue Staining and Data Collection

3.1. Tissue Staining

For the identification of cancerous cells, the prostate tissue was sectioned with a thickness of 4μm. The process of deparaffinization (i.e., removal of paraffin wax from slides prior to staining) is especially important after tissue sectioning because, otherwise, only poor staining may be achieved. However, in practice, each tissue section was deparaffinized and rehydrated in an appropriate manner and H&E staining was carried out successfully using an automated stainer (Autostainer XL, Leica). Hematoxylin and Eosin are positively and negatively charged, respectively. The nucleic acids in the nucleus are negatively charged components of basophilic cells; hematoxylin reacts with these components. Amino groups in proteins in the cytoplasm are positively charged components of acidophilic cells; eosin reacts with these components [46–48]. Figure 1 shows the visualization of the H&E stained biopsy image, which was analyzed using QuPath open-source software. The results of H&E staining are shown separately, with their respective chemical formulas.

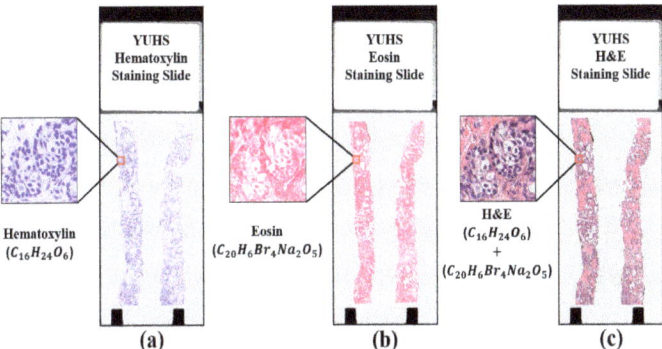

Figure 1. The visualization result of hematoxylin and eosin (H&E) staining slide. (**a**) Hematoxylin staining slide. (**b**) Eosin staining slide. (**c**) H&E staining slide obtained by combining (**a**,**b**). Note that the two slides (**a**,**b**) are highly dissimilar in texture, which is useful for analysis and classification.

3.2. Data Collection

The whole-slide H&E stained images of size 33,584 × 70,352 pixels were acquired from the pathology department of the Severance Hospital of Yonsei University. The slide images were further processed to generate multiple sizes (256 × 256, 512 × 512, and 1024 × 1024) of 2D patches by scanning at 40× optical magnification with 0.3NA objective using a digital camera (Olympus C-3000) which is attached to a microscope (Olympus BX-51). The extracted regions of interest (ROIs) were sent to the pathologist for prostate cancer (PCa) grading. Figure 2 shows an example of the cropped patches extracted from a whole-slide image. Regions containing background and adipose tissue were excluded. After the labeled patches were received, 6000 samples were selected, all with size 256 × 256 pixels (24 bit/pixel); the samples were divided equally into two classes: cancerous and non-cancerous. The tissue samples used in our research were extracted from 10 patients. These samples had an RGB color coding scheme (8 bits each for red, green, and blue).

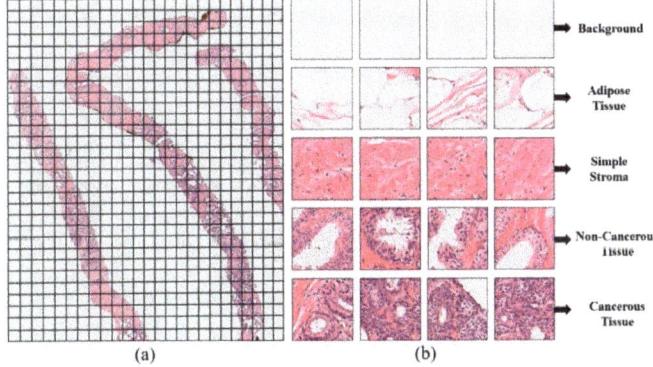

Figure 2. Data preparation of a sample histopathology slide from a prostatectomy. (**a**) An example of a whole-slide image where a sliding window method was applied to generate patch images. (**b**) The cropped patches obtained from (**a**) corresponded to the lowest and highest Gleason pattern, from well-differentiated to poorly differentiated, respectively. Among all patches in (**b**), the simple stroma, benign and malignant patches were selected for PCa analysis and classification.

4. Materials and Methods

4.1. Proposed Pipeline

Image and feature classification based on DL and ML methods showed some promising results in categorizing microscopic images of benign or malignant tissues. Our proposed pipeline for this paper is shown in Figure 3. Our analysis of a tissue image dataset was carried out in five phases, which include image pre-processing, analyze CNN models, feature analysis, model classification, and performance evaluation. In this study, we developed two LWCNN models (model 1 and model 2) and used state-of-art pre-trained models to carry out 2D image classification and perform a comparative analysis among the models. Also, EML classification was performed to classify the handcrafted (OCLBP and IOCLBP) and non-handcrafted (CNN-based) colour texture features extracted from tissue images.

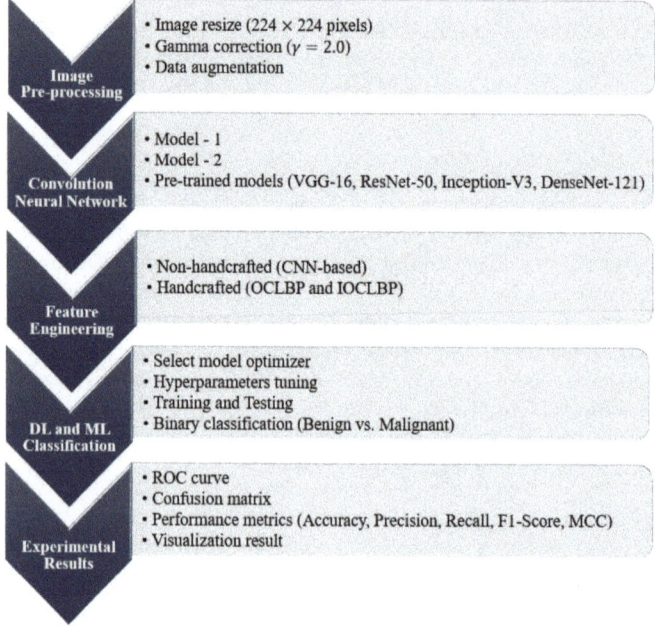

Figure 3. Proposed pipeline for image and feature classification based on a lightweight convolutional neural network (LWCNN) and ensemble machine learning (EML). LR: logistic regression, RF: random forest.

4.2. Image Preprocessing

In this phase, the preprocessing was carried out, whereby we resized the patches to 224 × 224 pixels for CNN training, and to adjust the contrast level of the image, power law (gamma) transformation [49,50] was applied to the resized images. The concept of gamma was used to encode and decode luminance values in image systems. Figure 4 illustrates the clarity of images before and after the application of this operation.

The dataset splitting was performed for training, validating, and testing the CNN models. The data samples were labeled with 0 (non-cancerous) and 1 (cancerous) for accurate classification and randomly assigned to one of three groups for training, validation, and testing, as shown in Table 1. The dataset used for DL and ML classification holds a total of 6000 samples. Out of these, 3600 were used for training, 1200 for validation, and 1200 for testing. Before the samples were fed to the network for classification, data augmentation was performed on the training set, which enabled analysis of model performance, reduction of overfitting problems, and improvement of generalization [51]. Therefore, to create some changes in the images, some transformations were applied using augmentation techniques, and these included rotation by 90°, transposition, random_brightening, and random_contrast, random_hue, and random_saturation, shown in Figure 5c,d. Keras and Tensorflow functions were used to execute data augmentation.

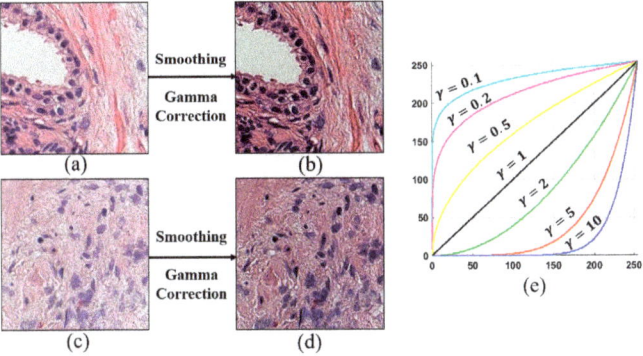

Figure 4. Image preprocessing using smoothing and gamma correction. (**a**,**c**) Original images of benign and malignant tissues, respectively. Here, the images are blurry and exhibit low contrast. (**b**,**d**) Images after removal of random noise, smoothing, and gamma correction. (**e**) Transformation curve for images with low and high contrast. Because the images in (**a**,**c**) have low contrast, $\gamma = 2$ was applied to adjust their intensities, obtaining images in (**b**,**d**) that appear clear and "fresh." Therefore, the tissue components were more visible after transformation, which was important for CNN classification.

Table 1. Assignment of benign and malignant samples into datasets for training, validation, and testing.

Dataset	Benign (0)	Malignant (1)	Total
Training	1800	1800	3600
Validation	600	600	1200
Testing	600	600	1200
Total	3000	3000	6000

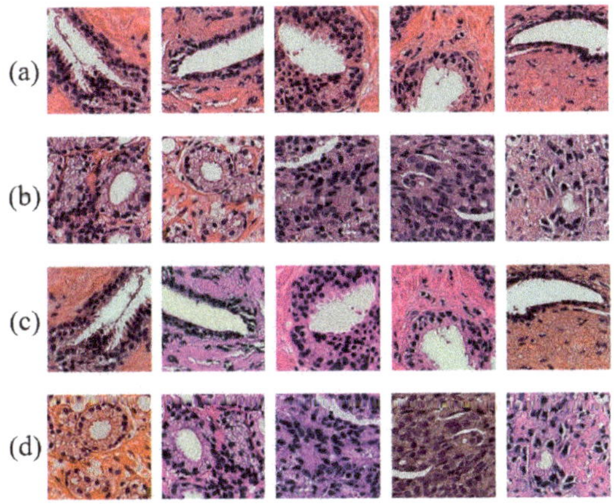

Figure 5. Randomly selected samples from the training dataset demonstrating data augmentation. (**a**,**b**) Images of benign and malignant tissues, respectively, before the transformation. (**c**,**d**) Transformed images from (**a**,**b**), respectively, after data augmentation.

4.3. Convolution Neural Network

To classify images of PCa, this paper introduces two LWCNN models to perform the classification of the GP and distinguish between two classes. Both model 1 and model 2 included CNN layers, such as those for input, convolution, rectified linear unit (ReLU), max pooling, dropout, flattening, GAP, and classification. Model 1 contained four convolutional blocks, with a depth of 10 layers, which interleaved two-dimensional (2D) convolutional layers (3 × 3 kernel, strides, and padding) with ReLU and batch normalization (BN) layers, followed by three max-pooling (2 × 2) and three dropout layers. To connect the neural network [52,53], a flattening layer and a sequence of three dense layers containing 1024, 1024, and 2 neurons were connected for feature classification and two probabilistic outputs. The sigmoid activation function [54,55] was used as a binary classifier. The numbers of filters in each block were 32, 64, 128, and 256. These filters acted as a sliding window over the entire image.

Model 2 contained three convolutional blocks, with a depth of seven layers, where the 2D convolutional, ReLU, and BN layers were identical to model 1 but were interleaved with two max-pooling (2 × 2) layers and one dropout layer. The numbers of convolutional filters in this model were 92, 192, and 384. A GAP layer was used instead of flattening, the classification section in this model also had three dense layers containing 64, 32, and 2 neurons. Here, a softmax [56,57] classifier was used to reduce binary loss. The input shape was set to 224 × 224 × 3 while building the model. The detailed design and specification of our lightweight CNN (LWCNN) models are shown in Figure 6 and Table 2, respectively. Model 2 was modified from model 1 based on multilevel feature analysis to improve classification accuracy and reduce validation loss, as shown in Figure 7.

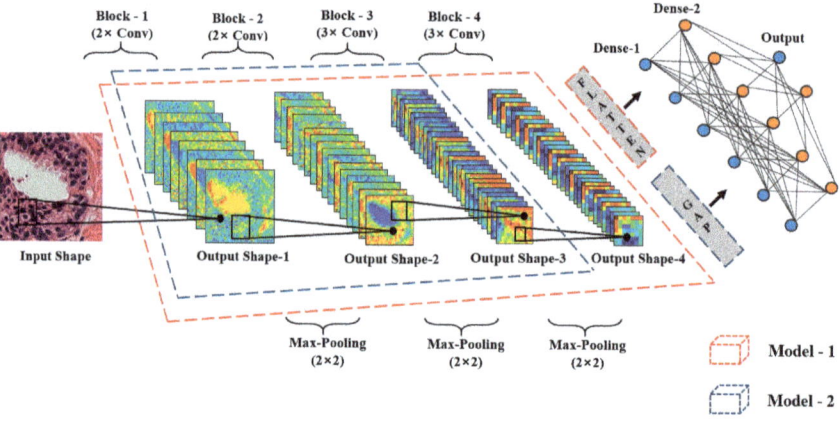

Figure 6. Structure of our lightweight convolutional neural networks for cancer image classification between two Gleason grade groups of prostate carcinoma. Spatial features are extracted from an image by convolving through one of the networks. Classification layers (flatten, global average pooling [GAP], dense-1, dense-2, and output) were used to find the required response based on features that were extracted by the convolutional neural network.

Table 2. Detailed information and specifications of lightweight convolutional neural network models. BN: batch normalization, GAP: global average pooling, ReLU: rectified linear unit.

	Layer Type	Filters	Output Shape	Kernel Size/Strides
	Model-1 Specification			
Input	Image	1	224 × 224 × 3	-
Block-1	2× convolutional + ReLU + BN	32	56 × 56 × 32	3 × 3/2
Block-2	2× convolutional + ReLU + BN	64	56 × 56 × 64	3 × 3/1

Table 2. Cont.

	Layer Type	Filters	Output Shape	Kernel Size/Strides
		Model-1 Specification		
-	Max pooling + dropout (0.25)	64	28 × 28 × 64	2 × 2/2
Block-3	3× convolutional + ReLU + BN	128	28 × 28 × 128	3 × 3/1
-	Max pooling + dropout (0.25)	128	14 × 14 × 128	2 × 2/2
Block-4	3× convolutional + ReLU + BN	256	14 × 14 × 256	3 × 3/1
-	Max pooling + dropout (0.25)	256	7 × 7 × 256	2 × 2/2
-	Flatten	-	12,544	-
-	Dense-1 + ReLU + BN	1024	1024	-
-	Dense-2 + ReLU + BN	1024	1024	-
-	Dropout (0.5)	1024	1024	-
Output	Sigmoid	2	2	-
		Model-2 specification		
Input	Image	1	224 × 224 × 3	-
Block-1	2× convolutional + ReLU + BN	92	56 × 56 × 92	5 × 5/2
Block-2	2× convolutional + ReLU + BN	192	56 × 56 × 192	3 × 3/1
-	Max pooling	192	28 × 28 × 192	2 × 2/2
Block-3	3× convolutional + ReLU + BN	384	28 × 28 × 384	3 × 3/1
-	Max pooling + dropout (0.25)	384	14 × 14 × 384	2 × 2/2
-	GAP	-	384	2 × 2/2
-	Dense-1 + ReLU + BN	64	64	-
-	Dense-2 + ReLU + BN	32	32	-
-	Dropout (0.5)	32	32	-
Output	Softmax	2	2	-

The multilevel feature maps were extracted after each convolutional block for pattern analysis and to understand the pixel distribution that the CNN detected, based on the number of convolution filters applied for edge detection and feature extraction. The convolution operation was performed by sliding the filter or kernel over the input image. Element-wise matrix multiplication was performed at each location in the image matrix and the output results were summed to generate the feature map. Max pooling was applied to reduce the input shape, prevent system memorization, and extract maximum information from each feature map. The feature maps from the first block held most of the information present in the image; that block acted as an edge detector. However, the feature map appeared more similar to an abstract representation and less similar to the original image, with advancement deeper into the network (see Figure 7). In block-3, the image pattern was somewhat visible, and by block-4, it became unrecognizable. This transformation occurred because deeper features encode high-level concepts, such as 2D information regarding the tissue (e.g., only spatial values of 0 or 1), while the CNN detects edges and shapes from low-level feature maps. Therefore, to improve the performance of the LWCNN, based on the observation that block-4 yielded unrecognizable images, model 2 was developed using three convolutional blocks, and selected as the model that this paper proposes.

To validate the performance of model 2 (LWCNN), we also included pre-trained CNN models (VGG-16, ResNet-50, Inceptio-V3, and DenseNet-121) for histopathology image classification. These models are very powerful and effective for extracting and classifying the deep CNN features. For each pre-trained network, the dense or classification block was configured according to the model specification. Sigmoid activation function was used for all the pre-trained models to perform binary classification.

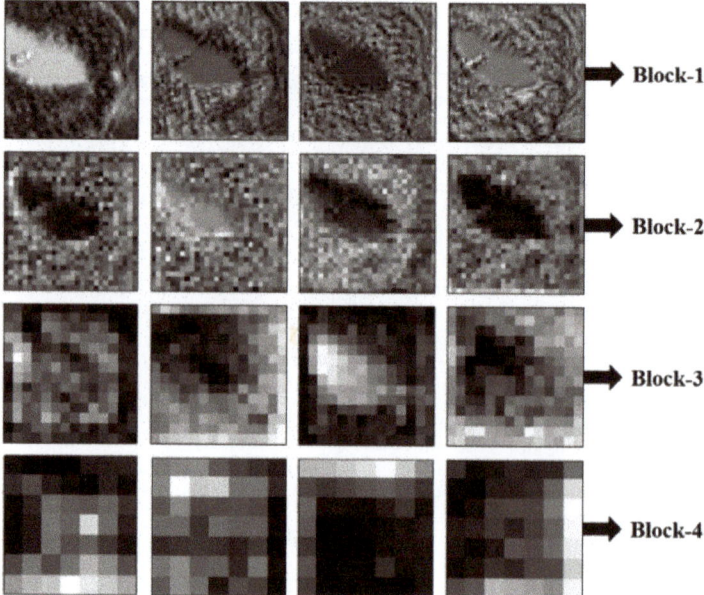

Figure 7. Multilevel feature map analysis for tissue image classification using a lightweight convolutional neural network. Visual analysis was performed by observing the pixel pattern in feature maps extracted from each block. Each block holds different information that is useful for convolutional neural network classification. Output shapes of feature maps from blocks 1–4 were: $56 \times 56 \times 92$, $28 \times 28 \times 192$, $14 \times 14 \times 384$, and $7 \times 7 \times 512$, respectively. Shown are four feature maps per block for the purpose of analysis, with 92, 192, 384, and 512 in each block, respectively. Analysis reveals that block-4 contains the maximum information regarding the image, but the resulting maps are less visually interpretable by people. With advancement deeper into the network, the feature maps become sparser, indicating that convolution filters detect fewer features. Therefore, block-4 was removed from model 2.

4.4. Feature Engineering

The extraction of texture features based on handcrafted and non-handcrafted was performed for ensemble machine learning (EML) classification. First, non-handcrafted or CNN-based features were extracted from the GAP layer of the proposed LWCNN (model 2). A different number of feature maps were generated from each CNN layer and the GAP mechanism was used to calculate the average value for each feature map. Second, a total of 20 handcrafted colour texture features were extracted using OCLBP and IOCLBP techniques. Out of these, 10 features were extracted using OCLBP, and 10 features using IOCLBP. The hand-designed feature analysis was performed for EML classification and compare with the non-handcrafted features classification results.

After we generate colour texture map, the LBP technique was applied to each colour channel (Red/Green/Blue) of OCLBP and IOCLBP separately. These state-of-art methods are the extensions of local binary patterns (LBP) and effective for colour image analysis. OCLBP and IOCLBP are the intra- and inter-channel descriptors with dissimilar local thresholding scheme (i.e., the peripheral pixels of OCLBP are thresholded at the central pixel value, and IOCLBP thresholding is based on the mean value) [30]. For each aforesaid state-of-art methods, the feature vector was obtained using general rotation-invariant operators (i.e., neighbor set of pixels p was placed on a circle of radius R) that can distinguish the spatial pattern and the contrast of local image texture. Therefore, the operators $p = 8$ and $R = 2$ were used to extract the colour features from the H&E stained tissue images.

4.5. DL and ML Classification

Prior to training and testing the LWCNN, pre-trained, and EML [58] models, we fine-tuned different types of parameters for better prediction and to minimize model loss. To compute the feature maps in each convolutional layer, a non-linear activation function (ReLU) was used, and the equation can be defined as:

$$A_{i,j,k} = \max(w_n^T I_{i,j} + b_n, 0) \tag{1}$$

where $A_{i,j,k}$ is the activation value of the nth feature map at the location (i, j), $I_{i,j}$ is the input patch, and w_n and b_n are the weight vector and bias term, respectively, of the nth filter.

BN was also used after each convolution layer to regularize the model, reducing the need for dropout. BN was used in our model because it is more effective than global data normalization. The latter normalization transforms the entire dataset so that it has a mean of zero and unit variance, while BN computes approximations of the mean and variance after each mini-batch. Therefore, BN enables the use of the ReLU activation function without saturating the model. Typically, BN is performed using the following equation:

$$BN(X_{normalize}) = (x_n - \mu_{mb}) / \sqrt{\sigma_{mb}^2 + c} \tag{2}$$

where x_n is the d-dimensional input, μ_{mb} and σ_{mb}^2 are the mean and variance, respectively, of the mini-batch, and c is a constant.

To optimize the weights of the network and analyze the performance of the LWCNN models, we performed a comparative analysis based on four different types of optimizers, namely stochastic gradient descent (SGD), Adadelta, Adam, and RMSprop. The results of comparative analysis are shown in the next section. The classification performance is measured using the cross-entropy loss, or log loss, whose output is a probability value between 0 and 1. To train our network, we used binary cross-entropy. The standard loss function for binary classification is given by:

$$Binary_{loss} = -\frac{1}{N} \sum_{i=1}^{N} [Y_i \times \log(M_w(X_i)) + (1 - Y_i) \times \log(1 - M_w(X_i))] \tag{3}$$

where N is the number of output class, X_i and Y_i are the input samples and target labels, respectively, and M_w is the model with network weight, w.

The hyperparameters were tuned while setting a minimum learning rate of 0.001 using the function known as ReduceLROnPlateau, a factor of 0.8 and patience of 10 were set; thus, if no improvement was observed in validation loss for 10 consecutive epochs, the learning rate was reduced by a factor of 0.8. The batch size was set to eight for training the model and regularization was applied by dropping out 25% and 50% of the weights in the convolution and dense blocks of LWCNN, respectively. The probabilistic output in the dense layer was computed using sigmoid and softmax classifiers.

In addition to CNN methods, traditional ML algorithms including logistic regression (LR) [59] and random forest (RF) [60] were used for features classification. In this paper, an ensemble voting method was proposed in which LR and RF classifiers were combined to create an EML model. This ensemble technique was used to classify the handcrafted and non-handcrafted features and compare the classification performance. The LWCNN, pre-trained, and EML models were tested using the unknown or unseen data samples. Typically, for ML classification, cross-validation was used by splitting the training data into k-fold (i.e., k = 5) to determine the model generalizability, and the result was computed by averaging the accuracies from each of the k trials. Prior to ML classification [61–63], the feature values for training and testing were normalized using the standard normal distribution function, which can be expressed as:

$$P_{i\_Normalised} = \frac{P_i - \mu}{\sigma} \tag{4}$$

where P_i is the *i*th pixel in an individual tissue image, and µ and σ are the mean and standard deviation of the dataset.

The DL and ML models were built with the Python 3 programming language using the Keras and Tensorflow libraries. Approximately 36 h were invested in fine-tuning the hyperparameters to achieve better accuracy. Figure 8 shows the entire process flow diagram for DL and ML classification. The hyperparameters that were used for DL and ML models are shown in Table 3.

The models were trained, validated, and tested on a PC with the following specifications: an Intel corei7 CPU (2.93 GHz), one NVIDIA GeForce RTX 2080 GPU, and 24 GB of RAM.

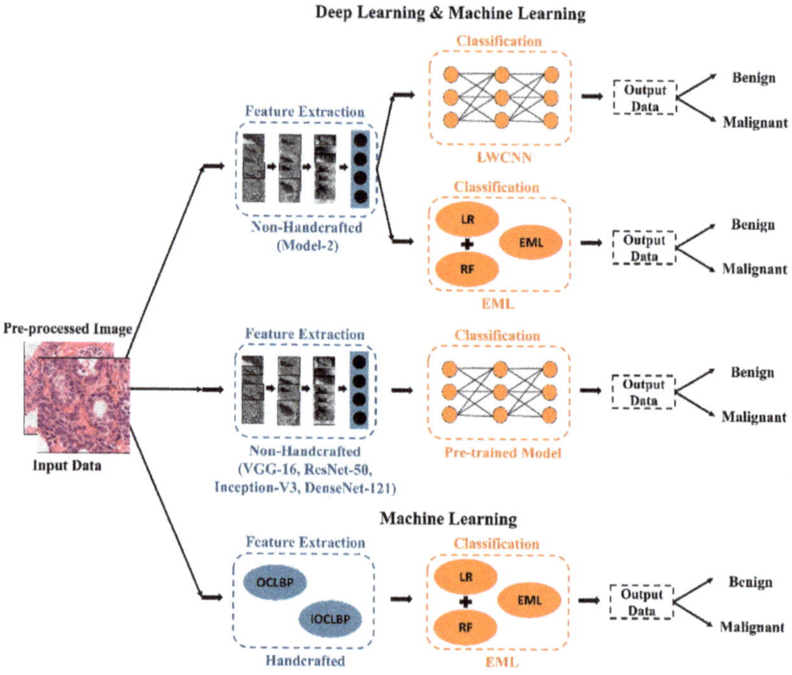

Figure 8. Flow diagram for DL and ML classification. Handcrafted and non-handcrafted colour texture descriptors were extracted for EML classification.

Table 3. Hyperparameters Tuning for DL and ML classifiers.

Models	Specification
Model-1, VGG-16, ResNet-50, Inception-V3, DenseNet-121	loss = binary_crossentropy; learning rate = start:1.0—auto reduce on plateau fraction: 0.8 after 10 consecutive non-declines of validation loss; classifier = sigmoid; epochs = 300
Model-2	loss = binary_crossentropy; learning rate = start:1.0—auto reduce on plateau fraction: 0.8 after 10 consecutive non-declines of validation loss; classifier = softmax; epochs = 300, kernel initializer = glorot_uniform
LR	C = 100, max_iter = 500, tol = 0.001, method = isotonic, penalty = l2
RF	n_estimators = 500, criterion = gini, max_depth = 9, min_samples_split = 5, min_samples_leaf = 4, method = isotonic

5. Experimental Results

This study mainly focuses on image classification based on AI. The proposed LWCNN (model 2) for tissue image classification and EML for feature classification produced reliable results, which met our requirements, at an acceptable speed. To develop DL models, a CNN approach was used as it is proven excellent performance in detecting specific regions for multiclass and binary classification. When splitting the dataset, a ratio of 8:2 was set for training and testing. Moreover, to validate the model after each epoch, the training set was further divided, such that 75% of the data was allocated for training and 25% was allocated for validation. Five-fold cross-validation was used during EML training. Algorithms used for preprocessing, data analysis, and classification were implemented in the MATLAB R2019a and PyCharm environments.

5.1. Performance Analysis

In this study, a binary classification approach was used to classify benign and malignant samples of prostate tissue. Two levels of classification were performed: DL (based on images) and ML (based on features). Table 4 shows the comparative analysis between the optimizers for model 1 and model 2, respectively. The developed LWCNN models were trained a couple of times by changing the optimizers during training.

Table 4. Comparison of the optimizers for tissue image classification.

Optimizers	Model-1		Model-2	
	Test Loss (%)	Test Accuracy (%)	Test Loss (%)	Test Accuracy (%)
SGD	0.51	85.7	0.25	93.3
RMSProp	1.00	85.5	0.62	89.3
Adam	0.45	84.4	0.28	91.1
Adadelta	0.54	89.1	0.25	94.0

From the above comparison table, we can analyze that the Adadelta performed the best and gave the best accuracies on test data for both the architectures. SGD and Adam performed close to Adadelta for model 2. On the other hand, RMSProp performed close to Adadelta for model 1. However, Adadelta (update version of Adam and Adagrad) is a more robust optimizer that restricts the window of accumulated past gradients to some fixed size w instead of accumulating all past square gradients. The comparison of these optimizers revealed that Aadelta is more stable and more rapid, hence, an overall improvement on SGD, RMSProp, and Adam. The behavior and performance of the optimizers were analyzed using the receiver operating characteristic (ROC) curve. It is a probabilistic curve that represents the diagnostic ability of a binary classifier system, including an indication of its effective threshold value. The area under the ROC curve (AUC) summarizes the extent to which a model can separate the two classes. Figure 9a,b show the ROC curve and corresponding AUC that depicts the effectiveness of different optimizers used for model 1 and model 2, respectively. For model 1, the AUCs were 0.95, 0.94, 0.96, and 0.93, and for model 2, 0.98, 0.97, 0.98, and 0.97 were obtained using Adadelta, RMSProp, SGD, and Adam, respectively.

Further, based on the optimum accuracy in Table 4, we carried out EML classification using the CNN extracted features from model 2, to analyze the efficiency of ML algorithms. Also, handcrafted features classification was performed to compare the performance with the non-handcrafted features classification results. Moreover, the EML model achieved promising results using the CNN-based features. Model 2 outperformed model 1 in overall accuracy, precision, recall, F1-score, and MCC, with values of 94.0%, 94.2%, 92.9%, 93.5%, and 87.0%, respectively. A confusion matrix (Figure 10) was generated based on the LWCNN model that yielded the optimum results, and thus most reliably distinguished malignant from benign tissue. Benign tissue was labeled as "0" and malignant was labeled as "1" to plot the confusion matrix for this binary classification. The four squares in the confusion matrix represent true positive, true negative, false positive, and false negative; their values were calculated using the test dataset based on the expected outcome and number of predictions of each class. Tables 5 and 6 show the overall comparative analysis for the DL and ML classification. The performance metrics used to evaluate the analysis results are accuracy, precision, recall, F1-score, and Matthews correlation coefficient (MCC).

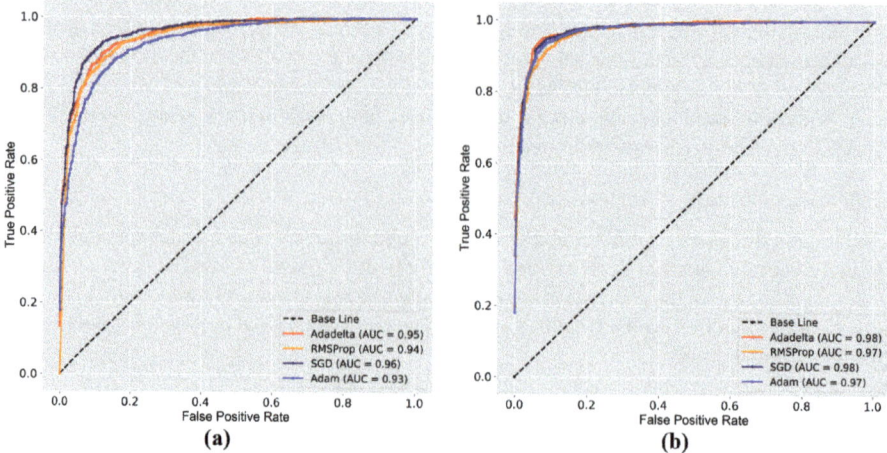

Figure 9. ROC curves for analyzing the behavior of different optimizers, generated by plotting predicted probability values (i.e., model's confidence scores). (**a**) Performance of model 1 based on sigmoid activation. (**b**) Performance of model 2 based on softmax activation function.

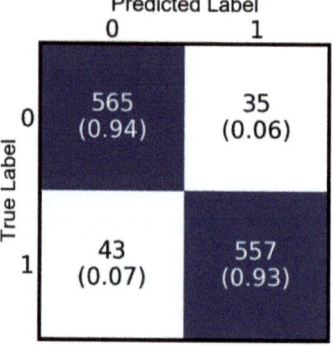

Figure 10. Confusion matrix of model 2, generated using the test dataset, showing results of binary classifications between benign (0) and malignant (1) tumors. Blue boxes at top-left and bottom-right represent true positive and true negative, respectively; white boxes at top-right and bottom-left represent false negative and false positive, respectively.

Table 5. Comparative analysis of lightweight and pre-trained CNN models based on non-handcrafted features. Metrics are for the test dataset.

	Deep Learning					
	Model-1	**Model-2**	**VGG-16**	**ResNet-50**	**Inception-V3**	**DenseNet-121**
Accuracy	89.1%	94.0%	92.0%	93.0%	94.6%	95.0%
Precision	89.2%	94.2%	92.2%	95.0%	96.5%	96.2%
Recall	89.1%	92.9%	91.9%	90.6%	93.2%	94.6%
F1-Score	89.0%	93.5%	92.0%	92.8%	94.8%	95.4%
MCC	78.3%	87.0%	84.0%	85.3%	89.5%	90.7%

Table 6. Comparative analysis of non-handcrafted and handcrafted features classification. Metrics are for the test dataset.

	Ensemble Machine Learning			
	CNN-Based	OCLBP	IOCLBP	OCLBP + IOCLBP
Accuracy	92.0%	69.3%	83.6%	85.0%
Precision	92.7%	66.0%	83.2%	85.5%
Recall	91.0%	70.6%	83.9%	84.5%
F1-Score	91.8%	68.2%	83.5%	85.0%
MCC	83.5%	38.6%	67.2%	69.8%

5.2. Visualization Results

The CAM technique was used to visualize the results from an activation layer (softmax) of the classification block. CAM is used to deduce which regions of an image are used by a CNN to recognize the precise class or group it contains [22,64]. Typically, it is difficult to visualize the results from hidden layers of a black box CNN model. More complexity is observed in feature maps with increasing depth in the network; thus, each image becomes increasingly abstract, encoding less information than the initial layers and appearing more blurred. Figure 11 shows the CAM results, indicating the method by which our DL network detected important regions; moreover, the network had learned a built-in mechanism to determine which regions merited attention. Therefore, this decision process was extremely useful in the classification network.

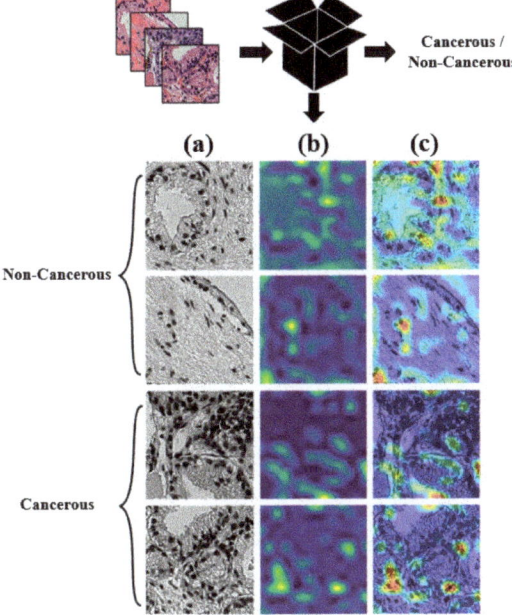

Figure 11. Class activation maps are extracted from one of the classification layers of our convolutional neural network. These show how images are classified and predicted by the neural network, although it is a black-box model. Top and bottom pairs of rows depict benign and malignant tissue images, respectively. (**a**) Input images with an RGB color scheme visualized as grayscale. (**b**) Activation map of classification block, showing detection of different regions in each tissue image. (**c**) Images overlaying (**a**,**b**), with spots indicating significant regions that the convolutional neural network used to identify a specific in that image.

Our CNN detected specific regions using the softmax classifier by incorporating spatially averaged information extracted by the GAP layer from the last convolution layer, which had an output shape of 14 × 14 × 384. The detected regions depicted in Figure 11c were generated by the application of a heat map to the CAM image in Figure 11b and overlaying that on the original image from Figure 11a. A heat map is highly effective for tissue image analysis; in this instance, it showed how the CNN detected each region of the image that is important for cancer classification. Doctors can use this information to better understand the classification (i.e., how the neural network predicted the presence of cancer in an image, based on the relevant regions). The visualization process was carried out using the test dataset, which was fed into the trained network of model 2.

In this study, supervised classification was performed for cancer grading, whereby our dataset was labeled with "0" and "1" to categorize benign and malignant tissue separately and independently. The probability distributions of data were similar in training and test sets, but the test dataset was independent of the training dataset. Therefore, after the model had been trained with several binary labeled cancer images, the unanalyzed dataset was fed to the network for accurate prediction between binary classes. Figure 12 shows examples of the binary classification results from our proposed model 2, with examples of images that were and were not predicted correctly. Notably, some images of benign were similar to malignant tissues and vice versa in terms of their nuclei distribution, intensity variation, and tissue texture. It was challenging for the model to correctly classify these images into the two groups.

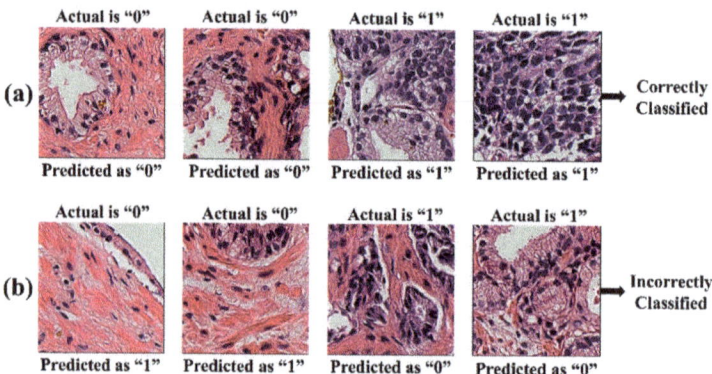

Figure 12. Cancer prediction using a binary labeled test dataset. Examples of images that were (a) correctly and (b) incorrectly classified, showing their actual and predicted labels.

6. Discussion

The main aim of this study was to develop LWCNN for benign and malignant tissue image classification based on multilevel feature map analysis and show the effectiveness of the model. Moreover, we developed an EML voting method for the classification of non-handcrafted (extracted from the GAP layer of model 2) and handcrafted (extracted using OCLBP and IOCLBP). Generally, in DL, the features are extracted automatically from raw data and further processed for classification using a neural network approach. However, for ML algorithms, features are extracted manually using different mathematical formulae; these are also regarded as handcrafted features. A CNN is suitable for complex detection tasks, such as analyses of scattered and finely drawn patterns in data. Of particular interest, in the malignant and benign classification task, model 2 was more effective than model 1. Indeed, model 1 performed below expectation, such that we modified it to improve performance, resulting in model 2. The modification comprised removal of the fourth convolutional block, flattening layer, and sigmoid activation function, as well as alterations of filter number and kernel size. Moreover, GAP replaced flattening after the third convolutional block, minimizing overfitting by reducing the total number of parameters in the model. The softmax activation function replaced the sigmoid activation function in the third dense layer. These modifications, based on the multilevel feature map analysis, improved the overall accuracy and localization ability of tissue image classification.

Furthermore, in this study, we have also compared our proposed CNN model with the well-known pre-trained models such as VGG-16, ResNet-50, Inception-V3, and DenseNet-121. Among these, DenseNet proved to give the highest accuracy of 95% followed by the Inception V3 with 94.6%. The pre-trained VGG-16 and ResNet-50 achieved 92% and 93%, respectively. Although DenseNet gained the highest accuracy among all the pre-trained models as well as our proposed model 2, it is not quite comparable with the motto of this paper. The ultimate goal of this paper was to develop a light-weighted CNN without a much-complicated structure with minimum possible convolutional layers and achieve better classification performance. Model 2 proved this hypothesis by achieving an overall accuracy of 94%. On the other hand, all the pre-trained models are well trained on a huge dataset (ImageNet) which includes 1000 classes. Therefore, it is evident that the classification of such models will be done accurately without much hassle. Nevertheless, the comparison of computational cost between the proposed LWCNN and other pre-trained models was performed to analyze the memory usage, trainable parameters, and learning (training and testing) time, shown in Table 7. First, according to the comparison Table 7, the number of trainable parameters used in the LWCNN model was reduced by more than 75% as compared to VGG-16, ResNet-50, and Inception-V3, and 2% as compared to DenseNet-121. Second, the memory usage of the proposed model was significantly less when compared to other models. Third, the time taken to train the proposed model was also drastically less. Among the pre-trained models, VGG-16 and ResNet-50 agree with the objective of this work. From Tables 5 and 7, it is evident that our LWCNN (model 2) is competitive and inexpensive, whereas, the state-of-art models were computationally expensive and achieved comparable results. Therefore, from this perspective, model 2 of our proposed work performed better than VGG-16 and ResNet-50 in terms of accuracy, besides employing a simple architecture.

Table 7. Comparing performance and computation cost of model-2 with other pre-trained models.

Models	Parameter (Trainable)	Model Memory Usage	Time to Solution (Minutes)	
			Train	Test
VGG-16	27,823,938	60.9 MB	570	<1
ResNet-50	23,538,690	148.4 MB	660	<1
Inception-V3	22,852,898	66.9 MB	600	<1
DenseNet-121	7,479,682	199.7 MB	700	<1
Model-2 (LWCNN)	5,386,638	44.7 MB	190	<1

Through fine-tuning of the hyperparameters, the CNN layers were determined to be optimal using the validation and test datasets. The modified, model 2 was adequate for the classification of benign and malignant tissue images. Our study examined the capability of the proposed LWCNN model to detect and forecast the histopathology images; a single activation map was extracted from each block (see Figure 13) to visualize the detection results using a heat map. Notably, we used an EML method for non-handcrafted and handcrafted features classification. However, the EML model was sufficiently powerful to classify the computational features extracted using the optimal LWCNN model, which predicted the samples of benign and malignant tissues almost perfectly accurately. Also, tissue samples that were classified and predicted using the softmax classifier are shown in quantile-quantile (Q–Q) plots of the prediction probability confidence for benign and malignant states in Figure 14a,b, respectively. These Q–Q plots allowed for the analysis of predictions. True and predicted probabilistic values were plotted according to true positive and true negative classifications of samples (see Figure 9), respectively.

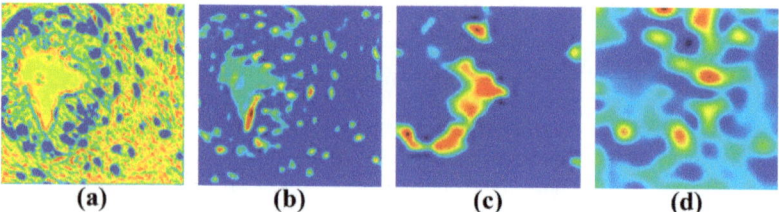

Figure 13. Visualizations of class activation maps generated from model 2, created using different numbers of filters. Outputs of (**a**) first convolutional, (**b**) second convolutional, (**c**) third convolutional, and (**d**) classification blocks. Colors indicate the most relevant regions for predicting the class of these histopathology images, as detected by the convolutional neural network.

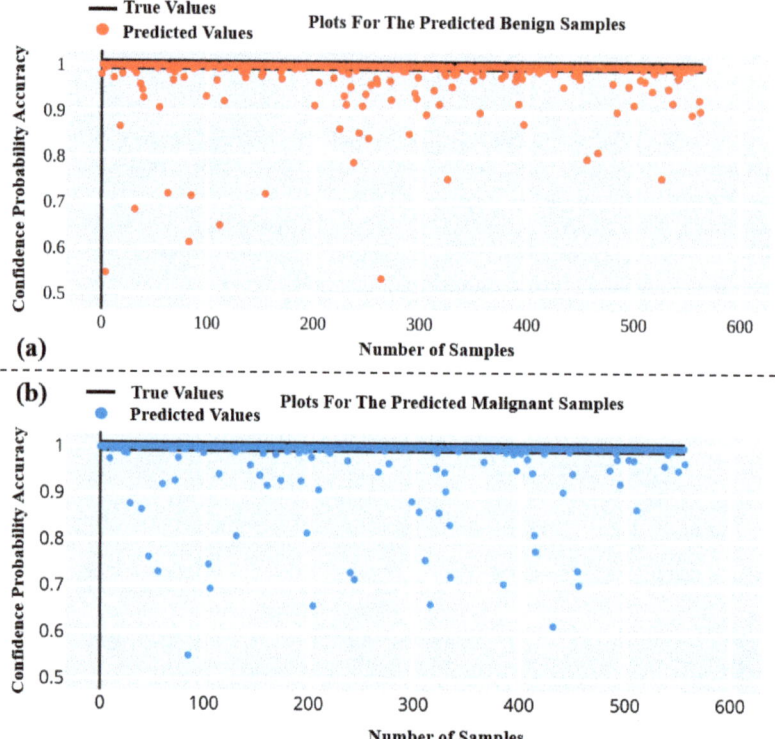

Figure 14. Quantile-quantile plot for true and predicted probabilistic values. (**a**) Samples that were benign and had true positive predictions. (**b**) Samples that were malignant and had true negative predictions.

In Q–Q plots, note that the black bar at the top parallel to the x-axis shows true probabilistic values; red (true positive) and blue (true negative) markers show the prediction confidence of each sample of a specific class. We used a softmax classifier, which normalizes the output of each unit to be between 0 and 1, ensuring that the probabilities always sum to 1. The number of samples used for each class was 600; the numbers correctly classified were 565 and 557 for true positive and true negative, respectively. A predicted probability value > 0.5 and <0.5 signifies an accurate classification and misclassification, respectively.

The combination of image-feature engineering and ML classification has shown remarkable performance in terms of medical image analysis and classification. In contrast, CNN adaptively learns various image features to perform image transformation, focusing on features that are highly predictive for a specific learning objective [65]. For instance, images of benign and malignant tissues could be presented to a network composed of convolutional layers with different numbers of filters that detect computational features and highlight the pixel pattern in each image. Based on these patterns, the network could use sigmoid and softmax classifiers to learn the extracted and important features, respectively. In DL, the "pipeline" of CNN's processing (i.e., from inputs to any output prediction) is opaque [66], performed automatically like a passage through a "black box" tunnel, where the user remains fully unaware of the process details. It is difficult to examine a CNN layer-by-layer. Therefore, each layer's visualization results and prediction mechanism are challenging to interpret.

Overall, all models performed well in tissue image classification, achieving comparable results. The EML method also worked well with CNN-extracted features, yielding comparable results. We conclude that, for image classification, models with very deep layers performed well by more accurately classifying the data samples. We aimed to build an LWCNN model with few feature-map layers and hyperparameters for prediction of cancer grading based on binary classification (i.e., benign vs. malignant). Our proposed methods have proven that lightweight models can achieve good results if the parameters are tuned appropriately. Furthermore, model 2 effectively recognized the histologic differences in tissue images and predicted their statuses with nearly perfect accuracy. The application of DL to histopathology is relatively new. However, it performs well and delivers accurate results. DL methods provide outstanding performance through black box layers; the outputs of each of these layers can be visualized using a heat map. In this study, our model provided insights into the histologic patterns present in each tissue image and can thus assist pathologists as a practical tool for analyzing tissue regions relevant to the worst prognosis. Heat map analyses suggested that the LWCNN can learn visual patterns of histopathological images containing different features relating to nuclear morphology, cell density, gland formation, and variations in the intensity of stroma and cytoplasm. Performance significantly improved when the first model was modified based on the feature map analysis.

7. Conclusions

In this study, 2D image classification was performed using PCa samples by leveraging non-handcrafted and handcrafted texture features to distinguish a malignant state of tissue from a benign state. We have presented LWCNN- and EML-based image and feature classification using feature map analysis. The DL models were designed with only a few CNN layers and trained with a small number of parameters. The computed feature maps of each layer were fed into these fully CNNs through the flattening and GAP layers, enabling binary classification using sigmoid and softmax classifiers. GAP and softmax were used for model 2, the optimal network in this paper. The GAP layer was used, instead of flattening, to minimize overfitting by reducing the total number of parameters in the model. This layer computes the mean value for each feature map, whereas flattening combined all feature maps extracted from the final convolution or pooling layers by changing the shape of the data from a 2D matrix of features into a one-dimensional array for passage to the fully CNN classifier. A comparative analysis was performed between the DL and EML classification results. Moreover, the computational cost was also compared among the models. The optimum LWCNN (i.e., model 2) and EML models (a combination of LR and RF classifiers) achieved nearly perfectly accurate results with significantly fewer trainable parameters. The proposed LWCNN model developed in the study achieved an overall accuracy of 94%, average precision of 94.2%, an average recall of 92.9%, an average f1-score of 93.5%, and MCC of 87%. On the other hand, using CNN-based features, the EML model achieved an overall accuracy of 92%, an average precision of 92.7%, an average recall of 91%, an average f1-score of 91.8%, and MCC of 83.5%.

To conclude, the analysis presented in this study is very encouraging. However, a model built for medical images may not work well for other types of images. There is a need to fine-tune the hyperparameters to control model overfitting and loss, thereby improving accuracy. The 2D LWCNN (model 2) developed in this study performed well, and therefore, the predicted true positive and true negative samples for benign and malignant, respectively, were plotted using Q-Q plots. The CAM technique was used to visualize the results of the block box CNN model. In the future, we will consider other methods and develop a more complex DL model and compare it with our optimal LWCNN model and other transfer learning models. Further, we will extend the research to multi-class classification (beyond binary) to simultaneously classify benign tissues, as well as grades 3–5.

Author Contributions: Funding acquisition, H.-K.C.; Methodology, S.B.; Resources, N.-H.C.; Supervision, H.-K.C.; Validation, H.-G.P.; Visualization, C.-H.K.; Writing—original draft, S.B.; Writing—review and editing, C.-H.K. and D.P. All authors have read and agreed to the published version of the manuscript.

Funding: This research was financially supported by the Ministry of Trade, Industry, and Energy (MOTIE), Korea, under the "Regional Specialized Industry Development Program (R&D, P0002072)" supervised by the Korea Institute for Advancement of Technology (KIAT).

Ethical Approval: All subjects' written informed consent waived for their participation in the study, which was approved by the Institutional Ethics Committee at College of Medicine, Yonsei University, Korea (IRB no. 1-2018-0044).

Conflicts of Interest: The authors declare that they have no conflicts of interest.

References

1. Siegel, R.L.; Miller, K.D.; Jemal, A. Cancer statistics, 2015. *CA Cancer J. Clin.* **2015**, *65*, 5–29. [CrossRef]
2. Chung, M.S.; Shim, M.; Cho, J.S.; Bang, W.; Kim, S.I.; Cho, S.Y.; Rha, K.H.; Hong, S.J.; Hong, C.-H.; Lee, K.S.; et al. Pathological Characteristics of Prostate Cancer in Men Aged <50 Years Treated with Radical Prostatectomy: A Multi-Centre Study in Korea. *J. Korean Med. Sci.* **2019**, *34*, 78. [CrossRef]
3. Yoo, S.; Gujrathi, I.; Haider, M.A.; Khalvati, F. Prostate Cancer Detection using Deep Convolutional Neural Networks. *Sci. Rep.* **2019**, *9*, 19518. [CrossRef]
4. Humphrey, P.A. Diagnosis of adenocarcinoma in prostate needle biopsy tissue. *J. Clin. Pathol.* **2007**, *60*, 35–42. [CrossRef]
5. Van Der Kwast, T.H.; Lopes, C.; Santonja, C.; Pihl, C.-G.; Neetens, I.; Martikainen, P.; Di Lollo, S.; Bubendorf, L.; Hoedemaeker, R.F. Guidelines for processing and reporting of prostatic needle biopsies. *J. Clin. Pathol.* **2003**, *56*, 336–340. [CrossRef] [PubMed]
6. Kim, E.H.; Andriole, G.L. Improved biopsy efficiency with MR/ultrasound fusion-guided prostate biopsy. *J. Natl. Cancer Inst.* **2016**, *108*. [CrossRef] [PubMed]
7. Heidenreich, A.; Bastian, P.J.; Bellmunt, J.; Bolla, M.; Joniau, S.; Van Der Kwast, T.; Mason, M.; Matveev, V.; Wiegel, T.; Zattoni, F.; et al. EAU Guidelines on Prostate Cancer. Part 1: Screening, Diagnosis, and Local Treatment with Curative Intent—Update 2013. *Eur. Urol.* **2014**, *65*, 124–137. [CrossRef] [PubMed]
8. Humphrey, P.A. Gleason grading and prognostic factors in carcinoma of the prostate. *Mod. Pathol.* **2004**, *17*, 292–306. [CrossRef]
9. Nagpal, K.; Foote, D.; Liu, Y.; Chen, P.-H.C.; Wulczyn, E.; Tan, F.; Olson, N.; Smith, M.C.; Mohtashamian, A.; Wren, J.H.; et al. Development and validation of a deep learning algorithm for improving Gleason scoring of prostate cancer. *NPJ Digit. Med.* **2019**, *2*, 48. [CrossRef]
10. Alqahtani, S.; Wei, C.; Zhang, Y.; Szewczyk-Bieda, M.; Wilson, J.; Huang, Z.; Nabi, G. Prediction of prostate cancer Gleason score upgrading from biopsy to radical prostatectomy using pre-biopsy multiparametric MRI PIRADS scoring system. *Sci. Rep.* **2020**, *10*, 7722. [CrossRef]
11. Zhu, Y.; Freedland, S.J.; Ye, D. Prostate Cancer and Prostatic Diseases Best of Asia, 2019: Challenges and opportunities. *Prostate Cancer Prostatic Dis.* **2019**, *23*, 197–198. [CrossRef] [PubMed]
12. Kumar, R.; Srivastava, R.; Srivastava, S.K. Detection and Classification of Cancer from Microscopic Biopsy Images Using Clinically Significant and Biologically Interpretable Features. *J. Med. Eng.* **2015**, *2015*, 457906. [CrossRef] [PubMed]

13. Cahill, L.C.; Fujimoto, J.G.; Giacomelli, M.G.; Yoshitake, T.; Wu, Y.; Lin, D.I.; Ye, H.; Carrasco-Zevallos, O.M.; Wagner, A.A.; Rosen, S. Comparing histologic evaluation of prostate tissue using nonlinear microscopy and paraffin H&E: A pilot study. *Mod. Pathol.* **2019**, *32*, 1158–1167. [CrossRef]
14. Otali, D.; Fredenburgh, J.; Oelschlager, D.K.; Grizzle, W.E. A standard tissue as a control for histochemical and immunohistochemical staining. *Biotech. Histochem.* **2016**, *91*, 309–326. [CrossRef] [PubMed]
15. Alturkistani, H.A.; Tashkandi, F.M.; Mohammedsaleh, Z.M. Histological Stains: A Literature Review and Case Study. *Glob. J. Health Sci.* **2015**, *8*, 72. [CrossRef] [PubMed]
16. Zarella, M.D.; Yeoh, C.; Breen, D.E.; Garcia, F.U. An alternative reference space for H&E color normalization. *PLoS ONE* **2017**, *12*, 0174489.
17. Lahiani, A.; Klaiman, E.; Grimm, O. Enabling histopathological annotations on immunofluorescent images through virtualization of hematoxylin and eosin. *J. Pathol. Inform.* **2018**, *9*, 1. [CrossRef] [PubMed]
18. Gavrilovic, M.; Azar, J.C.; Lindblad, J.; Wählby, C.; Bengtsson, E.; Busch, C.; Carlbom, I.B. Blind Color Decomposition of Histological Images. *IEEE Trans. Med. Imaging* **2013**, *32*, 983–994. [CrossRef]
19. Bautista, P.A.; Yagi, Y. Staining Correction in Digital Pathology by Utilizing a Dye Amount Table. *J. Digit. Imaging* **2015**, *28*, 283–294. [CrossRef]
20. Bianconi, F.; Kather, J.N.; Reyes-Aldasoro, C.C. Evaluation of Colour Pre-Processing on Patch-Based Classification of H&E-Stained Images. In *Digital Pathology. ECDP*; Lecture Notes in Computer Science; Springer: Cham, Switzerland, 2019; Volume 11435, pp. 56–64. [CrossRef]
21. Diamant, A.; Chatterjee, A.; Vallières, M.; Shenouda, G.; Seuntjens, J. Deep learning in head & neck cancer outcome prediction. *Sci. Rep.* **2019**, *9*, 2764.
22. Yamashita, R.; Nishio, M.; Do, R.K.G.; Togashi, K. Convolutional neural networks: An overview and application in radiology. *Insights Imaging* **2018**, *9*, 611–629. [CrossRef] [PubMed]
23. Sahiner, B.; Pezeshk, A.; Hadjiiski, L.; Wang, X.; Drukker, K.; Cha, K.H.; Summers, R.M.; Giger, M.L. Deep learning in medical imaging and radiation therapy. *Med. Phys.* **2019**, *46*, e1–e36. [CrossRef] [PubMed]
24. Nanni, L.; Ghidoni, S.; Brahnam, S. Handcrafted vs. non-handcrafted features for computer vision classification. *Pattern Recognit.* **2017**, *71*, 158–172. [CrossRef]
25. Lundervold, A.S.; Lundervold, A. An overview of deep learning in medical imaging focusing on MRI. *Z. Med. Phys.* **2019**, *29*, 102–127. [CrossRef] [PubMed]
26. Lee, J.-G.; Jun, S.; Cho, Y.-W.; Lee, H.; Kim, G.B.; Seo, J.B.; Kim, N. Deep Learning in Medical Imaging: General Overview. *Korean J. Radiol.* **2017**, *18*, 570–584. [CrossRef] [PubMed]
27. Bi, W.L.; Hosny, A.; Schabath, M.B.; Giger, M.L.; Birkbak, N.J.; Mehrtash, A.; Allison, T.; Arnaout, O.; Abbosh, C.; Dunn, I.F.; et al. Artificial intelligence in cancer imaging: Clinical challenges and applications. *CA Cancer J. Clin.* **2019**, *69*, 127–157. [CrossRef]
28. Jha, S.; Topol, E.J. Adapting to Artificial Intelligence. *JAMA* **2016**, *316*, 2353–2354. [CrossRef] [PubMed]
29. Badejo, J.A.; Adetiba, E.; Akinrinmade, A.; Akanle, M.B. Medical Image Classification with Hand-Designed or Machine-Designed Texture Descriptors: A Performance Evaluation. In *Internatioanl Conference on Bioinformatics and Biomedical Engineering*; Springer: Cham, Switzerland, 2018; pp. 266–275. [CrossRef]
30. Bianconi, F.; Bello-Cerezo, R.; Napoletano, P. Improved opponent color local binary patterns: An effective local image descriptor for color texture classification. *J. Electron. Imaging* **2017**, *27*, 011002. [CrossRef]
31. Kather, J.N.; Bello-Cerezo, R.; Di Maria, F.; Van Pelt, G.W.; Mesker, W.E.; Halama, N.; Bianconi, F. Classification of Tissue Regions in Histopathological Images: Comparison Between Pre-Trained Convolutional Neural Networks and Local Binary Patterns Variants. In *Intelligent Systems Reference Library*; Springer: Cham, Switzerland, 2020; pp. 95–115. [CrossRef]
32. Khairunnahar, L.; Hasib, M.A.; Bin Rezanur, R.H.; Islam, M.R.; Hosain, K. Classification of malignant and benign tissue with logistic regression. *Inform. Med. Unlocked* **2019**, *16*, 100189. [CrossRef]
33. Guidotti, R.; Monreale, A.; Ruggieri, S.; Turini, F.; Giannotti, F.; Pedreschi, D. A Survey of Methods for Explaining Black Box Models. *ACM Comput. Surv.* **2019**, *51*, 93. [CrossRef]
34. Hayashi, Y. New unified insights on deep learning in radiological and pathological images: Beyond quantitative performances to qualitative interpretation. *Inform. Med. Unlocked* **2020**, *19*, 100329. [CrossRef]
35. Lo, S.-C.; Lou, S.-L.; Lin, J.-S.; Freedman, M.; Chien, M.; Mun, S. Artificial convolution neural network techniques and applications for lung nodule detection. *IEEE Trans. Med. Imaging* **1995**, *14*, 711–718. [CrossRef] [PubMed]

36. Lo, S.-C.B.; Chan, H.-P.; Lin, J.-S.; Li, H.; Freedman, M.T.; Mun, S.K. Artificial convolution neural network for medical image pattern recognition. *Neural Netw.* **1995**, *8*, 1201–1214. [CrossRef]
37. LeCun, Y.; Bottou, L.; Bengio, Y.; Haffner, P. Gradient-based learning applied to document recognition. *Proc. IEEE* **1998**, *86*, 2278–2324. [CrossRef]
38. Liu, S.; Zheng, H.; Feng, Y.; Li, W. Prostate cancer diagnosis using deep learning with 3D multiparametric MRI. In *Medical Imaging 2017: Computer-Aided Diagnosis*; SPIE 10134; International Society for Optics and Photonics: Orlando, FL, USA, 2017; p. 1013428.
39. Han, Z.; Wei, B.; Zheng, Y.; Yin, Y.; Li, K.; Li, S. Breast Cancer Multi-classification from Histopathological Images with Structured Deep Learning Model. *Sci. Rep.* **2017**, *7*, 4172. [CrossRef]
40. Abraham, B.; Nair, M.S. Automated grading of prostate cancer using convolutional neural network and ordinal class classifier. *Inform. Med. Unlocked* **2019**, *17*, 100256. [CrossRef]
41. Truki, T. An Empirical Study of Machine Learning Algorithms for Cancer Identification. In Proceedings of the 2018 IEEE 15th International Conference on Networking, Sensing and Control (ICNSC), Zhuhai, China, 27–29 March 2018; pp. 1–5.
42. Veta, M.M.; Pluim, J.P.W.; Van Diest, P.J.; Viergever, M.A. Breast Cancer Histopathology Image Analysis: A Review. *IEEE Trans. Biomed. Eng.* **2014**, *61*, 1400–1411. [CrossRef]
43. Moradi, M.; Mousavi, P.; Abolmaesumi, P. Computer-Aided Diagnosis of Prostate Cancer with Emphasis on Ultrasound-Based Approaches: A Review. *Ultrasound Med. Biol.* **2007**, *33*, 1010–1028. [CrossRef]
44. Alom, Z.; Yakopcic, C.; Nasrin, M.S.; Taha, T.M.; Asari, V.K. Breast Cancer Classification from Histopathological Images with Inception Recurrent Residual Convolutional Neural Network. *J. Digit. Imaging* **2019**, *32*, 605–617. [CrossRef]
45. Wang, C.; Shi, J.; Zhang, Q.; Ying, S. Histopathological image classification with bilinear convolutional neural networks. In Proceedings of the 2017 39th Annual International Conference of the IEEE Engineering in Medicine and Biology Society (EMBC), Seogwipo, Korea, 15–16 July 2017; Volume 2017, pp. 4050–4053.
46. Smith, S.A.; Newman, S.J.; Coleman, M.P.; Alex, C. Characterization of the histologic appearance of normal gill tissue using special staining techniques. *J. Vet. Diagn. Investig.* **2018**, *30*, 688–698. [CrossRef]
47. Vodyanoy, V.; Pustovyy, O.; Globa, L.; Sorokulova, I. Primo-Vascular System as Presented by Bong Han Kim. *Evid. Based Complement. Altern. Med.* **2015**, *2015*, 361974. [CrossRef] [PubMed]
48. Larson, K.; Ho, H.H.; Anumolu, P.L.; Chen, M.T. Hematoxylin and Eosin Tissue Stain in Mohs Micrographic Surgery: A Review. *Dermatol. Surg.* **2011**, *37*, 1089–1099. [CrossRef] [PubMed]
49. Huang, S.-C.; Cheng, F.-C.; Chiu, Y.-S. Efficient Contrast Enhancement Using Adaptive Gamma Correction With Weighting Distribution. *IEEE Trans. Image Process.* **2012**, *22*, 1032–1041. [CrossRef] [PubMed]
50. Rahman, S.; Rahman, M.; Abdullah-Al-Wadud, M.; Al-Quaderi, G.D.; Shoyaib, M. An adaptive gamma correction for image enhancement. *EURASIP J. Image Video Process.* **2016**, *2016*, 35. [CrossRef]
51. Shorten, C.; Khoshgoftaar, T.M. A survey on Image Data Augmentation for Deep Learning. *J. Big Data* **2019**, *6*, 60. [CrossRef]
52. Lecun, Y.; Bengio, Y.; Hinton, G. Deep learning. *Nature* **2015**, *521*, 436–444. [CrossRef]
53. Kieffer, B.; Babaie, M.; Kalra, S.; Tizhoosh, H.R. Convolutional neural networks for histopathology image classification: Training vs. Using pre-trained networks. In Proceedings of the 2017 Seventh International Conference on Image Processing Theory, Tools and Applications (IPTA), Montreal, QC, Canada, 28 November–1 December 2017; pp. 1–6.
54. Mourgias-Alexandris, G.; Tsakyridis, A.; Passalis, N.; Tefas, A.; Vyrsokinos, K.; Pleros, N. An all-optical neuron with sigmoid activation function. *Opt. Express* **2019**, *27*, 9620–9630. [CrossRef]
55. Elfwing, S.; Uchibe, E.; Doya, K. Sigmoid-weighted linear units for neural network function approximation in reinforcement learning. *Neural Netw.* **2018**, *107*, 3–11. [CrossRef]
56. Kouretas, I.; Paliouras, V. Simplified Hardware Implementation of the Softmax Activation Function. In Proceedings of the 2019 8th International Conference on Modern Circuits and Systems Technologies (MOCAST), Thessaloniki, Greece, 13–15 May 2019; pp. 1–4.
57. Zhu, Q.; He, Z.; Zhang, T.; Cui, W. Improving Classification Performance of Softmax Loss Function Based on Scalable Batch-Normalization. *Appl. Sci.* **2020**, *10*, 2950. [CrossRef]
58. Dietterich, T.G. Ensemble Methods in Machine Learning. In *International Workshop on Multiple Classifier System*; Springer: Berlin, Heidelberg, 2000; pp. 1–15. [CrossRef]

59. Dikaios, N.; Alkalbani, J.; Sidhu, H.S.; Fujiwara, T.; Abd-Alazeez, M.; Kirkham, A.; Allen, C.; Ahmed, H.; Emberton, M.; Freeman, A.; et al. Logistic regression model for diagnosis of transition zone prostate cancer on multi-parametric MRI. *Eur. Radiol.* **2015**, *25*, 523–532. [CrossRef]
60. Nguyen, C.; Wang, Y.; Nguyen, H.N. Random forest classifier combined with feature selection for breast cancer diagnosis and prognostic. *J. Biomed. Sci. Eng.* **2013**, *6*, 551–560. [CrossRef]
61. Cruz, J.A.; Wishart, D.S. Applications of Machine Learning in Cancer Prediction and Prognosis. *Cancer Inform.* **2006**, *2*, 59–77. [CrossRef]
62. Tang, T.T.; Zawaski, J.A.; Francis, K.N.; Qutub, A.A.; Gaber, M.W. Image-based Classification of Tumor Type and Growth Rate using Machine Learning: A preclinical study. *Sci. Rep.* **2019**, *9*, 12529. [CrossRef] [PubMed]
63. Madabhushi, A.; Lee, G. Image analysis and machine learning in digital pathology: Challenges and opportunities. *Med. Image Anal.* **2016**, *33*, 170–175. [CrossRef] [PubMed]
64. Yang, W.; Huang, H.; Zhang, Z.; Chen, X.; Huang, K.; Zhang, S. Towards Rich Feature Discovery With Class Activation Maps Augmentation for Person Re-Identification. In Proceedings of the 2019 IEEE/CVF Conference on Computer Vision and Pattern Recognition (CVPR), Long Beach, CA, USA, 15–20 June 2019; pp. 1389–1398.
65. Hou, X.; Gong, Y.; Liu, B.; Sun, K.; Liu, J.; Xu, B.; Duan, J.; Qiu, G. Learning Based Image Transformation Using Convolutional Neural Networks. *IEEE Access* **2018**, *6*, 49779–49792. [CrossRef]
66. Chai, X.; Gu, H.; Li, F.; Duan, H.; Hu, X.; Lin, K. Deep learning for irregularly and regularly missing data reconstruction. *Sci. Rep.* **2020**, *10*, 3302. [CrossRef]

Publisher's Note: MDPI stays neutral with regard to jurisdictional claims in published maps and institutional affiliations.

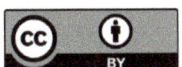

© 2020 by the authors. Licensee MDPI, Basel, Switzerland. This article is an open access article distributed under the terms and conditions of the Creative Commons Attribution (CC BY) license (http://creativecommons.org/licenses/by/4.0/).

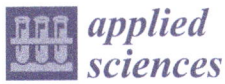

Article

Simulation Study of Low-Dose Sparse-Sampling CT with Deep Learning-Based Reconstruction: Usefulness for Evaluation of Ovarian Cancer Metastasis

Yasuyo Urase [1], Mizuho Nishio [1,2,*], Yoshiko Ueno [1], Atsushi K. Kono [1], Keitaro Sofue [1], Tomonori Kanda [1], Takaki Maeda [1], Munenobu Nogami [1], Masatoshi Hori [1] and Takamichi Murakami [1]

1. Department of Radiology, Kobe University Graduate School of Medicine, 7-5-2 Kusunoki-cho, Chuo-ku, Kobe 650-0017, Japan; y.urase220@gmail.com (Y.U.); yoshiu0121@gmail.com (Y.U.); ringonotegami@mac.com (A.K.K.); keitarosofue@yahoo.co.jp (K.S.); k_a@hotmail.co.jp (T.K.); maetaka@med.kobe-u.ac.jp (T.M.); aznogami@med.kobe-u.ac.jp (M.N.); horimsts@med.kobe-u.ac.jp (M.H.); murataka@med.kobe-u.ac.jp (T.M.)
2. Department of Diagnostic Imaging and Nuclear Medicine, Kyoto University Graduate School of Medicine, 54 Kawahara-cho, Shogoin, Sakyo-ku, Kyoto 606-8507, Japan
* Correspondence: nmizuho@med.kobe-u.ac.jp; Tel.: +81-78-382-6104; Fax: +81-78-382-6129

Received: 11 May 2020; Accepted: 24 June 2020; Published: 28 June 2020

Abstract: The usefulness of sparse-sampling CT with deep learning-based reconstruction for detection of metastasis of malignant ovarian tumors was evaluated. We obtained contrast-enhanced CT images (n = 141) of ovarian cancers from a public database, whose images were randomly divided into 71 training, 20 validation, and 50 test cases. Sparse-sampling CT images were calculated slice-by-slice by software simulation. Two deep-learning models for deep learning-based reconstruction were evaluated: Residual Encoder-Decoder Convolutional Neural Network (RED-CNN) and deeper U-net. For 50 test cases, we evaluated the peak signal-to-noise ratio (PSNR) and structural similarity (SSIM) as quantitative measures. Two radiologists independently performed a qualitative evaluation for the following points: entire CT image quality; visibility of the iliac artery; and visibility of peritoneal dissemination, liver metastasis, and lymph node metastasis. Wilcoxon signed-rank test and McNemar test were used to compare image quality and metastasis detectability between the two models, respectively. The mean PSNR and SSIM performed better with deeper U-net over RED-CNN. For all items of the visual evaluation, deeper U-net scored significantly better than RED-CNN. The metastasis detectability with deeper U-net was more than 95%. Sparse-sampling CT with deep learning-based reconstruction proved useful in detecting metastasis of malignant ovarian tumors and might contribute to reducing overall CT-radiation exposure.

Keywords: deep learning; neoplasm metastasis; ovarian neoplasms; radiation exposure; tomography; x-ray computed

1. Introduction

Ovarian cancer is the eighth leading cause of female cancer death worldwide [1]. The incidence of ovarian cancer increases with age and peaks in the 50s [2]. In addition, malignant germ cell tumors are common in young patients with ovarian cancer [3].

CT is the major modality for diagnosing ovarian tumors, detecting metastases, staging ovarian cancer, following up after surgery, and assessing the efficacy of chemotherapy. On the other hand, CT radiation exposure may be associated with elevated risks of thyroid cancer and leukemia in all adult ages and non-Hodgkin lymphoma in younger patients [4]. Patients with ovarian cancer tend to be relatively young, therefore the reduction of CT radiation exposure is essential. Radiation exposure of CT is mainly controlled by adjusting the tube current and voltage [5]. Lowering the radiation dose increases image noise, so techniques that reduce image noise and artifacts and maintain image quality are needed. Low-dose CT images were reconstructed by filtered back projection (FBP) until the 2000s. However, iterative reconstruction (IR) has been the mainstream since the first IR technique was clinically introduced in 2009 [5]. IR reconstruction technology has evolved into hybrid IR, followed by model-based IR (MBIR). IR has been reported to reduce the radiation dose by 23–76% without compromising image quality compared to FBP [5].

In recent years, a technique called sparse-sampling CT that resembles compressed sensing in MRI has attracted attention as a possible new technique to reduce exposure. This technique reconstructs CT images using a combination of sparse-sampling CT and Artificial intelligence (AI), especially deep learning, which may reduce CT radiation exposure more than two-fold over the current technology [5]. A few studies show that with the application of sparse-sampling CT and deep-learning, lower-dose CT could be used [6,7].

Research for the noise reduction of CT images using deep learning started around 2017 [6–15]. In 2017, image-patch-based noise reduction was performed using deep learning model on low-dose CT images [7,11]. On the other hand, Jin et al. show that entire CT images could be directly denoised using U-net [9]. To improve perceptual image quality, generative adversarial network (GAN) was introduced for CT noise reduction [12,13]. Following the advancement in noise reduction using deep learning, Nakamura et al. evaluated noise reduction using deep learning on a real CT scanner [16]. However, most of them focused on quantitative measures such as peak signal-to-noise ratio (PSNR) and structural similarity (SSIM). To the best of our knowledge, there are few studies that radiologists visually evaluate abnormal lesions such as metastasis on CT images processed with deep learning [16]. Furthermore, the quantitative measure, such as PSNR and SSIM, and human perceived quality were not always consistent in agreement [17]. Therefore, we suggest that PSNR and SSIM alone cannot assure clinical usefulness and accuracy of lesion detection.

The present study aimed to evaluate the usefulness of sparse-sampling CT with deep learning-based reconstruction for radiologists to detect the metastasis of malignant ovarian tumors. This study used both quantitative and qualitative assessment of denoised sparse-sampling CT with deep learning, including PSNR and SSIM, along with radiologists' visual score, and the detectability of metastasis.

2. Materials and Methods

This study used anonymized data from a public database. The regulations of our country did not require approval from an institutional review board for the use of a public database.

2.1. Dataset

Our study tested abdominal CT images obtained from The Cancer Imaging Archive (TCIA) [18–20]. We used one public database of the abdominal CT images available from TCIA: The Cancer Genome Atlas Ovarian Cancer (TCGA-OV) dataset. The dataset is constructed by a research community of The Cancer Genome Atlas, which focuses on the connection between cancer phenotypes and genotypes by providing clinical images. In TCGA-OV, clinical, genetic, and pathological data reside in Genomic Data Commons Data Portal while radiological data are stored on TCIA.

TCGA-OV provides 143 cases of abdominal contrast-enhanced CT images. Two cases were excluded from the current study because the pelvis was outside the CT scan range. The other 141 cases were included in the current study. The 141 cases were randomly divided into 71 training cases, 20 validation cases, and 50 test cases. For training, validation, and test cases, the number of CT images was 6916, 1909, and 4667, respectively.

2.2. Simulation of Sparse-Sampling CT

As in a previous study [9], sparse-sampling CT images were simulated for the 141 sets of abdominal CT images of TCGA-OV. The original CT images of the TCGA-OV were converted into sinograms with 729 pixels by 1000 views using ASTRA-Toolbox (version 1.8.3, https://www.astra-toolbox.com/), an open-source MATLAB and Python toolbox of high-performance graphics processing unit (GPU) primitives for two- and three-dimensional tomography [21,22]. To simulate sparse-sampling CT images, we uniformly (at regular view intervals) subsampled the sinograms by a factor of 10, which corresponded to 100 views. While a 20-fold subsampling rate was used in the previous study [9], our preliminary analysis revealed that the abdominal CT images simulated with a 20-fold subsampling rate were too noisy. As a result, we utilized a 10-fold subsampling rate in the current study. The 10-fold subsampled sinograms were converted into the sparse-sampling CT images using FBP of the ASTRA-Toolbox.

2.3. Deep Learning Model

To denoise the sparse-sampling CT images, a deep learning model was employed in the current study. The outline of the training phase and deployment (denoising) phase using a deep learning model is represented in Figure 1. In the training phase, pairs of original and noisy CT images were used for constructing a deep learning model. In the deployment phase, we used the deep learning model for denoising noisy CT images. We used a workstation with GPU (GeForce RTX 2080 Ti with 11 GB memory, NVIDIA Corporation, Santa Clara, California, USA) for training and denoising.

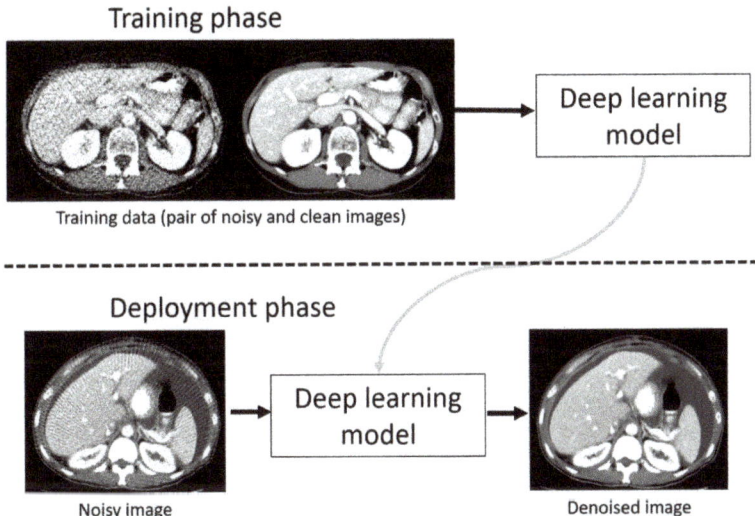

Figure 1. Outline of the training phase and deployment phase of the deep learning model.

Two types of deep learning models were evaluated: Residual Encoder-Decoder Convolutional Neural Network (RED-CNN) [7] and deeper U-net with skip connection [6]. RED-CNN combines autoencoder, deconvolution network, and shortcut connections into its network structure, and it performed well in denoising low-dose CT images. RED-CNN used image patches extracted from the CT image (size 55 × 55 pixels) for training [7]. Nakai et al. developed deeper U-net for denoising sparse-sampling chest CT images and showed that deeper U-net was superior to conventional U-net with skip connection [6]. Contrary to RED-CNN, deeper U-net made it possible to use entire CT images (size 512 × 512 pixels) as training data. In the current study, the usefulness of deeper U-net was evaluated and compared to RED-CNN.

We implemented deeper U-net using Keras (version 2.2.2, https://keras.io/) with TensorFlow (version 1.10.1, https://www.tensorflow.org/) backend. The major differences of network structure between our deeper U-net and Nakai's deeper U-net were as follows: (i) the number of maxpooling and upsampling was 9; (ii) the numbers of feature maps in the first convolution layer of our U-net was 104. After the maxpooling layer, the number of feature maps in the convolution layer was doubled. However, if the numbers of feature maps were 832, the number of feature maps was not increased even after the maxpooling layer. The changes in the network structure of our deeper U-net including (i) and (ii) are shown in Appendix A in more detail. To train deeper U-net, pairs of original CT images and sparse-sampling CT images were prepared. Mean squared error (MSE) between the original and denoised CT images represented the loss function of deeper U-net. Adam was used as an optimizer, and its learning rate was 0.0001. The number of training epochs was 100. 4000 seconds were required for training deeper U-net per one epoch.

RED-CNN was trained using its PyTorch implementation (https://github.com/SSinyu/RED_CNN). RED-CNN was trained on an image patch size of 55 × 55 pixels. Network-related parameters of RED-CNN were retained as described previously [7].

2.4. Quantitative Image Analysis

To evaluate the denoising performance of deep learning models, we used two quantitative measures, PSNR and SSIM, on the 4667 CT images from 50 test cases [23]. These parameters are frequently used as standard objective distortion measures and for quantitative assessment of the reconstructed images [10]. PSNR is defined as

$$PSNR = 20 log_{10}(\frac{MAX_I}{\sqrt{MSE}}), \quad (1)$$

where MSE is calculated between the denoised and original CT images, and MAX_I is the maximum value of the original CT image. SSIM is a metric that supposedly reflects the human visual perception rather than PSNR. It is defined as

$$SSIM(x,y) = \frac{(2u_x u_y + c_1)(2s_{xy} + c_2)}{(u_x^2 + u_y^2 + c_1)(s_{x2} + s_{y2} + c_2)}, \quad (2)$$

where x and y are the denoised and original CT images, respectively; u_x and u_y are the means of x and y, respectively; s_{x2} and s_{y2} are the variances of x and y, respectively; s_{xy} is the covariance of x and y; and c_1 and c_2 are determined by the dynamic range of the pixel values to stabilize the division with the weak denominator. Scikit-image (version 0.13.0, https://scikit-image.org/) was used to calculate these two quantitative measures.

2.5. Qualitative Image Analysis

On the denoised sparse-sampling CT of 50 test cases, the normal and abnormal lesions were visually evaluated. For the qualitative evaluation, four radiologists were participated, two performing visual assessments as readers and the other two defining and extracting lesions to be assessed. The two groups were independent of each other.

As readers, two board-certified radiologists (with 17 and 10 years of experience, respectively) independently evaluated the denoised CT images and referred to the original images on 3D Slicer (version 4.10.2, https://www.slicer.org/) [24]. For all visual evaluations described in the following section, we used a five-point scale as follows: (1) Unacceptable, (2) Poor, (3) Moderate, (4) Good, and (5) Excellent. The definition of each score and detail procedure of qualitative evaluation is shown in Tables 1–3 and Appendix B, respectively.

Table 1. Score criteria for entire CT image quality.

Score		
(A) Overall Image Quality		
1	Unacceptable	non-diagnostic
2	Poor	poor visualization, heavily blurred appearance of structures
3	Moderate	moderate visualization, moderate blurring
4	Good	good delineation, slight blurring
5	Excellent	excellent visualization, sharp delineation (equivalent to or better compared with the original image)
(B) Noise and Artifacts		
1	Unacceptable	heavily noise and artifacts, structures are not visible on entire CT image
2	Poor	heavily noise and artifacts, structures are not visible on most parts of CT image
3	Moderate	moderate noise and artifacts, but acceptable for clinical evaluation
4	Good	minor, but slight noticeable noise and artifacts are found compared with the original image
5	Excellent	noise and artifacts levels are equivalent to or better compared with the original image

Table 2. Score criteria for the evaluation of normal local lesions (common iliac artery, internal iliac artery, and external iliac artery).

Score		
1	Unacceptable	Unrecognizable
2	Poor	recognizable, but not measurable
3	Moderate	recognizable and measurable despite a blurred margin
4	Good	slightly blurry margin compared with the original image, but measurable
5	Excellent	measurable, sharp margin equivalent to the original image

Table 3. Score criteria for the evaluation of abnormal lesions.

Score		
1	Unacceptable	unrecognizable
2	Poor	recognizable but unqualified for diagnosis and measurement
3	Moderate	moderately noisy and blurry, but recognizable and qualified for diagnosis and measurement
4	Good	qualified for diagnosis and measurement, but slightly inferior to the original image
5	Excellent	qualified for diagnosis and measurement equivalent to the original image

The image quality evaluation of the entire CT and the normal local lesions were evaluated. For the entire CT image quality, (A) Overall image quality and (B) Noise and artifacts were evaluated. The overall image quality represented a comprehensive evaluation, including noise, artifacts, and visibility of anatomical structures.

As an evaluation of the normal local lesions, the visibility of the iliac artery (the common iliac artery, internal iliac artery, and external iliac artery) was evaluated. A score was given on whether or not the diameter could be reliably measured at each of the three points of the common iliac artery, internal iliac artery, and external iliac artery.

Peritoneal dissemination, liver metastasis, and lymph node metastasis were visually evaluated as abnormal lesions by the two radiologists. The abnormal lesions were determined by the consensus of two other independent board-certified radiologists (6 and 14 years of experience, respectively) on the original CT image based on the following criteria. Peritoneal dissemination was defined as previously established as either 1) an isolated mass or 2) subtle soft tissue infiltration and reticulonodular lesions [25]. Lymph node metastasis was defined as short axis ≥10 mm. With reference to RESIST v1.1, we defined peritoneal dissemination and liver metastasis as follows: peritoneal dissemination for non-measurable or measurable (long axis ≥ 10 mm); liver metastasis (long axis ≥ 10 mm) [26]. The measurable lesions of peritoneal dissemination were further subdivided into long axis ≤ 20 and > 20 mm because the staging of FIGO 2014 differs depending on the size [27].

2.6. Statistical Analysis

For the quantitative assessment of the denoised images, the mean scores of PSNR and SSIM of deeper U-net and RED-CNN were calculated. All the qualitative image quality scores were compared between deeper U-net and RED-CNN using the Wilcoxon signed-rank test. For each abnormal lesion, a 5-point score ≥ 3 was regarded as true positive (TP), and a 5-point score < 3 as false negative (FN). He detectability of abnormal lesions was calculated based on the following equation: $\frac{TP}{TP+FN}$ (sensitivity). The detectability of abnormal lesions was compared between deeper U-net and RED-CNN using the McNemar test. Statistical analyses were performed using JMP® (version 14.2, SAS Institute Inc., Cary, NC, USA). All tests were two sided with a significance level of 0.05.

3. Results

A summary of patient demographics of the 141 cases is provided in Table 4. The location of ovarian cancer and clinical stage were available from TCIA in 140 cases. Age was obtained from DICOM data of CT images. For the 50 test cases, 124 abnormal lesions were determined, including 6 liver metastases, 25 lymph node metastases, and 93 peritoneal disseminations. For the peritoneal disseminations, the numbers of non-measurable lesions, measurable lesions with long axis $\leq$ 20 mm, and measurable lesions with long axis > 20 mm were 53, 28, and 12, respectively.

For normal local lesions and abnormal lesions, representative images of the original CT and denoised CT obtained using deeper U-net and RED-CNN are shown in Figure 2. Additionally, representative images of the original CT, the sparse-sampled CT images before denoised processing and denoised CT obtained using deeper U-net and RED-CNN are shown in Figure 3.

Table 4. Patient demographics of TCGA-OV.

Category		Value
Age *		60.7 ± 11.2 (39–82)
Location of tumor		
	Bilateral	107
	Left	13
	Right	12
	Not available	8
Clinical Stage **		
	IB	1
	IC	7
	IIA	3
	IIB	1
	IIC	4
	IIIA	1
	IIIB	3
	IIIC	93
	IV	26
	Not available	1

Note: * and ** indicate that data were obtained from 139 and 140 cases, respectively. Clinical stage of patients were extracted from the TCGA-OV dataset; it is unknown whether the clinical stage is based on FIGO classification or TNM classification.

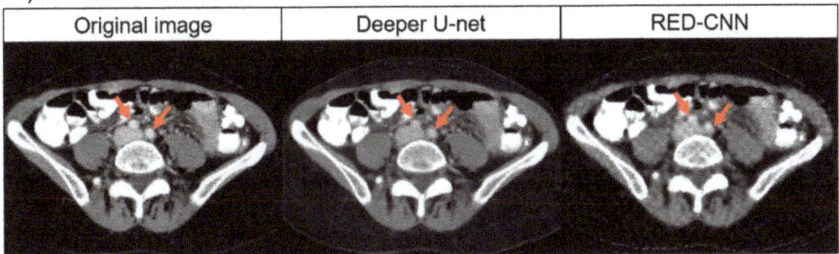
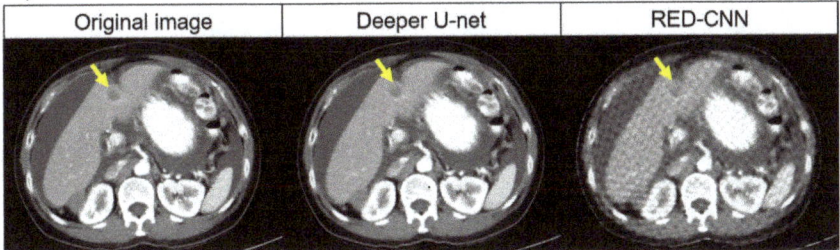

Figure 2. Representative images of the original CT and denoised CT obtained using deeper U-net and RED-CNN. Note: (**A**) Visual scores of common iliac artery (red arrow): 5 points for deeper U-net, 2 points for RED-CNN for reader 1; 4 points for deeper U-net, 2 points for RED-CNN for reader 2. (**B**) Visual scores of liver metastasis (yellow arrow): 3 points for deeper U-net, 2 points for RED-CNN for reader 1; 4 points for deeper U-net, 2 points for RED-CNN for reader 2. Abbreviation: RED-CNN, Residual Encoder-Decoder Convolutional Neural Network.

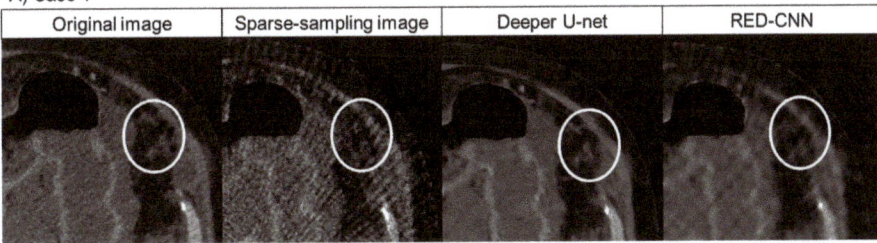
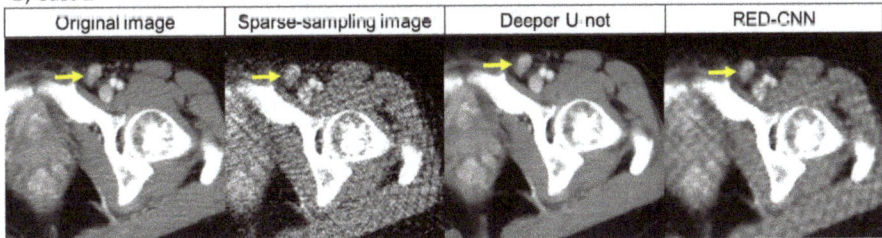

Figure 3. *Cont.*

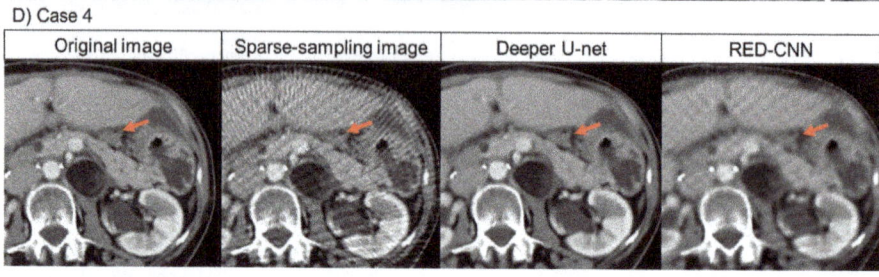

Figure 3. Representative images of the original CT, sparse-sampling CT before denoising, and denoised CT obtained using deeper U-net and RED-CNN. Note: (**A**) Case 1: Visual scores of peritoneal dissemination (white circle): 4 points for deeper U-net, 1 points for RED-CNN for reader 1; 4 points for deeper U-net, 1 points for RED-CNN for reader 2. (**B**) Case 2: Visual scores of lymph node metastasis (yellow arrow): 5 points for deeper U-net, 2 points for RED-CNN for reader 1; 4 points for deeper U-net, 2 points for RED-CNN for reader 2. (**C**) Case 3: Visual scores of liver metastasis (red arrow): 4 points for deeper U-net, 2 points for RED-CNN for reader 1; 4 points for deeper U-net, 2 points for RED-CNN for reader 2. (**D**) Case 4: Visual scores of peritoneal dissemination (red arrow): 4 points for deeper U-net, 2 points for RED-CNN for reader 1; 4 points for deeper U-net, 1 points for RED-CNN for reader 2.

3.1. Quantitative Image Analysis

We evaluate the PSNR and SSIM on the 4667 CT images from 50 test cases. The number of samples for calculating PSNR and SSIM was 4667. The PSNR and SSIM were 29.2 ± 1.49 and 0.75 ± 0.04 for the sparse-sampling images before denoising, 48.5 ± 2.69 and 0.99 ± 0.01 for deeper U-net, and 37.3 ± 1.97 and 0.93 ± 0.02 for RED-CNN.

3.2. Qualitative Image Analysis

The results of the visual evaluation are shown in Figures 4 and 5 and Tables 5 and 6. For all items of the visual evaluation, deeper U-net scored better than that of RED-CNN for both readers as shown in Table 7.

Streak artifacts tended to be stronger on images at the upper abdomen level, especially where the lung and abdominal organs were visualized on the same image.

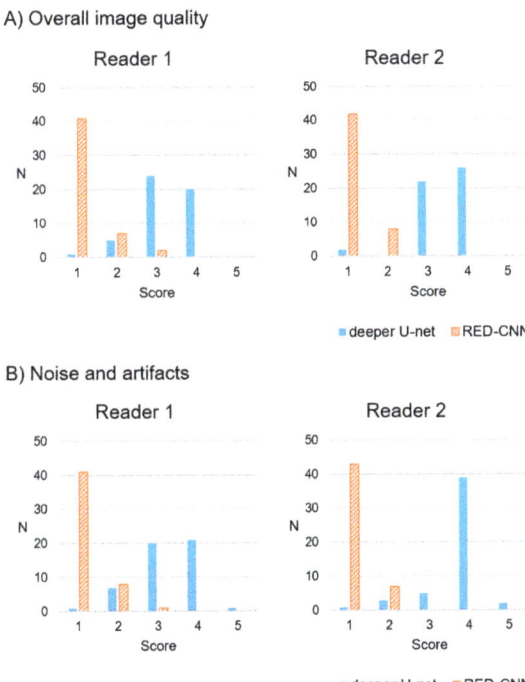

Figure 4. Visual evaluation of entire CT image quality by the two readers using different deep learning algorithms.

Table 5. Visual evaluation of entire CT image quality by the two readers using different deep learning algorithms.

(A) Overall Image Quality					
	Reader 1			Reader 2	
score	Deeper U-net	RED-CNN	score	Deeper U-net	RED-CNN
1	1	41	1	2	42
2	5	7	2	0	8
3	24	2	3	22	0
4	20	0	4	26	0
5	0	0	5	0	0
(B) Noise and Artifacts					
	Reader 1			Reader 2	
score	Deeper U-net	RED-CNN	score	Deeper U-net	RED-CNN
1	1	41	1	1	43
2	7	8	2	3	7
3	20	1	3	5	0
4	21	0	4	39	0
5	1	0	5	2	0

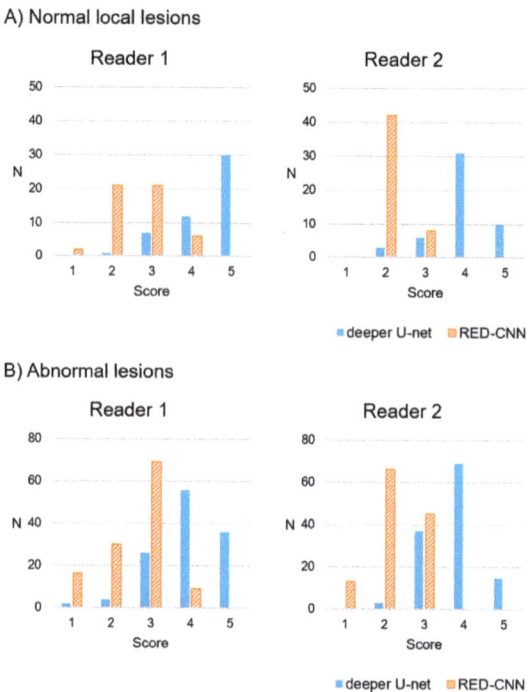

Figure 5. Visual evaluation of normal local lesions and abnormal lesions by the two readers using different deep learning algorithms.

Table 6. Visual evaluation of normal local lesions and abnormal lesions by the two readers using different deep learning algorithms.

	(A) Normal Local Lesions				
	Reader 1			Reader 2	
score	Deeper U-net	RED-CNN	score	Deeper U-net	RED-CNN
1	0	2	1	0	0
2	1	21	2	3	42
3	7	21	3	6	8
4	12	6	4	31	0
5	30	0	5	10	0
	(B) Abnormal Lesions				
	Reader 1			Reader 2	
score	Deeper U-net	RED-CNN	score	Deeper U-net	RED-CNN
1	2	16	1	13	0
2	6	30	2	66	5
3	26	69	3	44	35
4	56	9	4	0	68
5	34	0	5	0	15

Table 7. Results of visual evaluations by the two readers using different deep learning algorithms.

		Deeper U-net	RED-CNN	p
Entire CT image quality				
(A) Overall image quality	Reader 1	median, 3; IQR, 3 to 4	median, 1; IQR, 1 to 1	<0.0001
	Reader 2	median, 4; IQR, 3 to 4	median, 1; IQR, 1 to 1	<0.0001
(B) Noise and artifacts	Reader 1	median, 3; IQR, 3 to 4	median, 1; IQR, 1 to 1	<0.0001
	Reader 2	median, 4; IQR, 4 to 4	median, 1; IQR, 1 to 1	<0.0001
Normal local lesions	Reader 1	median, 5; IQR, 4 to 5	median, 3; IQR, 2 to 3	<0.0001
	Reader 2	median, 4; IQR, 4 to 4	median, 2; IQR, 2 to 2	<0.0001
Abnormal lesions	Reader 1	median, 4; IQR, 3 to 5	median, 3; IQR, 2 to 3	<0.0001
	Reader 2	median, 4; IQR, 3 to 4	median, 2; IQR, 2 to 3	<0.0001

Abbreviation: IQR, interquartile range; RED-CNN, Residual Encoder-Decoder Convolutional Neural Network.

The detectability of abnormal lesions with deeper U-net was significantly better than that with RED-CNN: 95.2% (118/124) vs. 62.9% (78/124) ($p < 0.0001$) for reader 1 and 97.6% (121/124) vs. 36.3% (45/124) ($p < 0.0001$) for reader 2. The number of FN with deeper U-net were six and three for readers 1 and 2, respectively. All these abnormal lesions were non-measurable peritoneal dissemination, which were identified as slight subtle soft-tissue infiltration and reticulonodular lesions on the original CT image. The representative images of the FN case are shown in Figure 6.

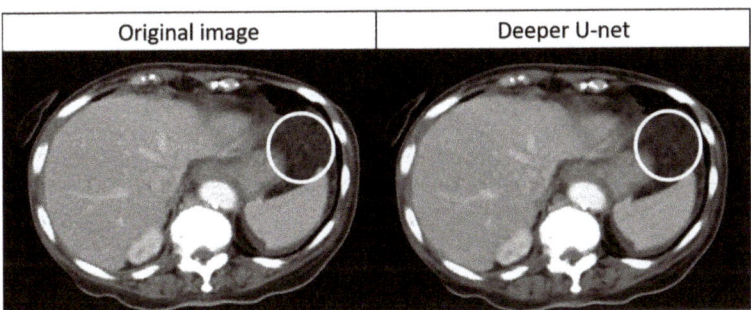

Figure 6. A representative undiagnosable lesion on denoised CT image with deeper U-net. Note: The circle shows non-measurable peritoneal dissemination. With deeper U-net, the score was 1 point for reader 1 and 2 points for reader 2.

4. Discussion

In the current study, we compared the quantitative and qualitative image quality of sparse-sampling CT denoised with deeper U-net and RED-CNN. RED-CNN was compared with our deeper U-net because of its similar network structure [7]. For quantitative analysis, mean scores of PSNR and SSIM of CT image quality with deeper U-net were better than those with RED-CNN. For all of the visual evaluation items, the scores of CT image quality with deeper U-net were significantly better than those of RED-CNN. In addition, the detectability of ovarian cancer metastasis was more than 95% in deeper U-net.

A few studies on deep learning-based reconstruction have shown that it improved image quality and reduced noise and artifacts better than hybrid IR and MBIR [8,16,28]. Nakamura et al. reported that deep learning reconstruction could reduce noise and artifacts more than hybrid IR could and that it may improve the detection of low-contrast lesions when evaluating hypovascular hepatic metastases [16]. While their study did not evaluate low-dose CT, the deep learning model is also considered an effective method with the potential to use lower-dose CT techniques such as sparse sampling with clinically acceptable results [5]. Our results showed that denoising with deeper U-net could be used to detect ovarian cancer metastasis.

To the best of our knowledge, this was the first study that evaluated the detectability of cancer metastasis, including peritoneal dissemination, liver metastasis, and lymph node metastasis on deep learning-based reconstructed CT images. The usefulness of sparse-sampling CT with deep learning has been previously reported [6,7,9,10], but image evaluation was limited to quantitative measures in most of these studies. While Nakai et al. reported on quantitative and qualitative assessments of the efficacy of deep learning on chest CT images [6], our study evaluated the usefulness of sparse-sampling CT denoised with deep learning techniques from the clinical viewpoint. We have proven that deeper U-net has an excellent ability to improve image quality and detectability of metastasis, and it could prove effective in clinical practice.

The performance difference between deeper U-net and RED-CNN was significant when assessing sparse-sampling CT images. A strong streak artifact around bony structures affected the image quality of sparse-sampling CT [29]. Therefore, to improve the image quality of sparse-sampling CT, an ideal deep learning model should reduce streak artifact associated with anatomical structures. RED-CNN used an image patch (size 55 × 55 pixels) for its training, therefore the algorithm had difficulty discerning between a streak artifact and anatomical structures. As a result, reducing the streak artifact related to anatomical structure may be limited in RED-CNN. In contrast, since deeper U-net used the entire CT image (size 512 × 512 pixels) for training, deeper U-net could be optimized to reduce streak artifact related to anatomical structures. This difference between the two deep learning models may lead to performance differences shown in the current study.

Since score 5 was defined as image quality and visualization equivalent to original CT (Tables 1–3), the denoised CT images of deeper U-net was not the same image quality as original CT images from the viewpoint of score. However, the visual scores and detectability of deeper U-net were sufficiently high.

Although patients with peritoneal dissemination are diagnosed as advanced stage, complete debulking surgery can be expected to improve the prognosis in epithelial malignant ovarian tumor [30]. In addition, there are some histological types with a favorable prognosis due to successful chemotherapy, such as yolk sac tumor [31]. Thus, the reduction of CT-radiation exposure is essential for patients with ovarian cancer. With our proposed method, theoretically, the CT radiation exposure can be reduced to one-tenth of that of the original CT. The reduction of radiation exposure may reduce the incidence of radiation-induced cancer. Furthermore, while we evaluated about only the detection of metastasis of malignant ovarian tumors in the current study, we speculate that the proposed method may be applied to other diseases.

While our results show that deeper U-net proved useful in detecting cancer metastasis, there were several drawbacks in the model. First, fine anatomical structures were obscured due to excessive denoising. This effect might be minimized by blending images of FBP and deep learning-based reconstruction, such as hybrid IR and MBIR, by adjusting radiation exposure (rate of sparse sampling) and blending rate. Secondly, the strong streak artifacts around the prosthesis and the upper abdomen compromised diagnostic ability near these anatomical lesions. Furthermore, streak artifacts tended to be stronger on images at the upper abdomen level, especially where the lung and abdominal organs were visualized on the same image. This effect may have resulted from the relatively small number of training data images that included both lung and abdominal organs compared to images that included only abdominal organs. Since ovarian cancer primarily metastasizes to the peritoneal liver surface and the liver, improving the image quality in these areas is considered a future research area. Increasing the number of training data images with cross-sections displaying both the lung and abdominal organs may help improve image quality and reduce streak artifacts in deep learning models, including deeper U-net.

Our study had several limitations. First, we used images from only one public database. The application of our deep learning model should be further evaluated in other databases. Second, sparse-sampling images cannot be obtained from real CT scanners at the current time. Our simulated subsampled images may differ from the images on real scanners. In future, we need to evaluate the performance of our deeper U-net using real CT acquisitions. Third, images obtained with the deep learning model of GAN tended to be more "natural" than those obtained with conventional deep learning model. However, the noise reduction of GAN is weaker than that of a conventional deep learning model [17]. There was a concern that the radiologist's ability to detect metastasis might decline if the noise reduction was insufficient. Therefore, GAN was not used in the current study. Finally, because of our study design, we did not evaluate false positives, true negatives, and specificity in the current study. Therefore, it is necessary to conduct radiologists' observer studies in which false positives and true negatives are evaluated.

5. Conclusions

Sparse-sampling CT with deep learning reconstruction could prove useful in detecting metastasis of malignant ovarian tumors and might contribute to reducing CT radiation exposure. With our proposed method, theoretically, the CT radiation exposure can be reduced to one-tenth of that of the original CT, while keeping the detectability of ovarian cancer metastasis more than 95%. It may reduce the incidence of radiation-induced cancer.

Author Contributions: Conceptualization, M.N. (Mizuho Nishio); methodology, M.N. (Mizuho Nishio); software, M.N. (Mizuho Nishio); validation, M.N. (Mizuho Nishio), Y.U. (Yasuyo Urase); formal analysis, Y.U. (Yasuyo Urase), M.N. (Mizuho Nishio); investigation, Y.U. (Yasuyo Urase), M.N. (Mizuho Nishio), Y.U. (Yoshiko Ueno), A.K.K.; resources, M.N. (Mizuho Nishio); data curation, M.N. (Mizuho Nishio); writing—original draft preparation, Y.U. (Yasuyo Urase); writing—review and editing, Y.U. (Yasuyo Urase), M.N. (Mizuho Nishio), Y.U. (Yoshiko Ueno), A.K.K., K.S., T.K., T.M. (Takaki Maeda), M.N. (Munenobu Nogami), M.H., T.M. (Takamichi Murakami); visualization, Y.U. (Yasuyo Urase), and M.N. (Mizuho Nishio); supervision, T.M. (Takamichi Murakami); project administration, M.N. (Mizuho Nishio); funding acquisition, M.N. (Mizuho Nishio). All authors have read and agreed to the published version of the manuscript.

Funding: This research was funded by the JSPS KAKENHI (Grant Number JP19K17232 and JP19H03599).

Acknowledgments: The authors would like to thank Izumi Imaoka from department of Radiology, Kobe Minimally invasive Cancer Center for her suggestion about defining metastatic lesions of ovarian cancer.

Conflicts of Interest: The authors declare no conflict of interest. The funders had no role in the design of the study; in the collection, analyses, or interpretation of data; in the writing of the manuscript, or in the decision to publish the results.

Appendix A. Network Structure of Deeper U-Net

The network structure of our deeper U-net is slightly modified from original deeper U-net [6]. The differences between the two networks were as follows:

1. The numbers of maxpooling and upsampling were 9 in our deeper U-net.
2. The numbers of feature maps in the first convolution layer of our U-net was 104. After the maxpooling layer, the number of feature maps in the convolution layer was doubled. However, if the numbers of feature maps were 832, the number of feature maps was not increased even after the maxpooling layer.
3. Rectified Linear Unit (ReLU) was used, instead of Leaky ReLU.
4. Probability of Dropout was changed. 0.2% was used in our deeper U-net.

Appendix B. Detail Procedure of Qualitative Evaluation by Radiologists

The detail procedure of qualitative evaluation was as follows. Two board-certified radiologists (17 and 10 years of experience, respectively) independently performed the visual evaluation as readers. The patient IDs of TCGA-OV in 50 test cases were sorted in alphabetical and numerical order, and the two radiologists interpreted the CT images in this order. All the 50 sets of denoised CT images with deeper U-net were evaluated first, then followed by those with RED-CNN. Image quality evaluation of the entire CT and the local normal lesions were performed by comparing the original image and the denoised image on 3D Slicer (version 4.10.2, https://www.slicer.org/) [24], and then the abnormal lesions were evaluated. Two other board-certified radiologists (6 and 14 years of experience, respectively) determined the abnormal lesions on the original image by consensus, and recorded the locations of the abnormal lesions on a file. In evaluating the abnormal lesions, the two readers referred to the file for the locations of abnormal lesions. At the time of interpretation, the two readers were informed of patient's age, and blind to all other clinical data. The image quality differed greatly between the two models, therefore the readers could easily determine the deep learning model with which the given CT images were denoised. Therefore, the interpretation order of the denoised images with deeper U-net and RED-CNN was not randomized. It was presumed that bias in evaluation of denoised CT images was inevitable even if interpretation order of deeper U-net and RED-CNN was randomized or the evaluations of CT images denoised with the two models were performed separately at long interval.

References

1. Ferlay, J.; Colombet, M.; Soerjomataram, I.; Mathers, C.; Parkin, D.M.; Piñeros, M.; Znaor, A.; Bray, F. Estimating the global cancer incidence and mortality in 2018: GLOBOCAN sources and methods. *Int. J. Cancer* **2019**, *144*, 1941–1953. [CrossRef]
2. Heints, A.; Odicino, F.; Maisonneuve, P.; Qiomm, M.A.; Benedet, J.L.; Creasman, W.T.; Ngan, H.Y.S.; Pecorelli, S.; Beller, U. Carcinoma of the ovary. *Int. J. Gynecol. Obstet.* **2006**, *95*, s161–s192. [CrossRef]
3. Webb, P.M.; Jordan, S.J. Epidemiology of epithelial ovarian cancer. *Best Pract. Res. Clin. Obstet. Gynaecol.* **2017**, *41*, 3–14. [CrossRef]
4. Shao, Y.-H.; Tsai, K.; Kim, S.; Wu, Y.-J.; Demissie, K. Exposure to Tomographic Scans and Cancer Risks. *JNCI Cancer Spectr.* **2019**, *4*, pkz072. [CrossRef] [PubMed]
5. Willemink, M.J.; Noël, P.B. The evolution of image reconstruction for CT—From filtered back projection to artificial intelligence. *Eur. Radiol.* **2019**, *29*, 2185–2195. [CrossRef] [PubMed]
6. Nakai, H.; Nishio, M.; Yamashita, R.; Ono, A.; Nakao, K.K.; Fujimoto, K.; Togashi, K. Quantitative and Qualitative Evaluation of Convolutional Neural Networks with a Deeper U-Net for Sparse-View Computed Tomography Reconstruction. *Acad. Radiol.* **2019**, *27*, 563–574. [CrossRef] [PubMed]
7. Chen, H.; Zhang, Y.; Kalra, M.K.; Lin, F.; Chen, Y.; Liao, P.; Member, S.; Wang, G. Low-Dose CT with a Residual Encoder-Decoder Convolutional Neural Network (RED-CNN). *IEEE Trans. Med. Imaging* **2017**, *36*, 2524–2534. [CrossRef]
8. Tatsugami, F.; Higaki, T.; Nakamura, Y.; Yu, Z.; Zhou, J.; Lu, Y.; Fujioka, C.; Kitagawa, T.; Kihara, Y.; Iida, M.; et al. Deep learning–based image restoration algorithm for coronary CT angiography. *Eur. Radiol.* **2019**, *29*, 5322–5329. [CrossRef]
9. Jin, K.H.; McCann, M.T.; Froustey, E.; Unser, M. Deep Convolutional Neural Network for Inverse Problems in Imaging. *IEEE Trans. Image Process.* **2017**, *26*, 4509–4522. [CrossRef]
10. Han, Y.; Ye, J.C. Framing U-Net via Deep Convolutional Framelets: Application to Sparse-View CT. *IEEE Trans. Med. Imaging* **2018**, *37*, 1418–1429. [CrossRef]
11. Nishio, M.; Nagashima, C.; Hirabayashi, S.; Ohnishi, A.; Sasaki, K.; Sagawa, T.; Hamada, M.; Yamashita, T. Convolutional auto-encoders for image denoising of ultra-low-dose CT. *Heliyon* **2017**, *3*, e00393. [CrossRef]
12. Kang, E.; Koo, H.J.; Yang, D.H.; Seo, J.B.; Ye, J.C. Cycle-consistent adversarial denoising network for multiphase coronary CT angiography. *Med. Phys.* **2019**, *46*, 550–562. [CrossRef]
13. Wolterink, J.M.; Leiner, T.; Viergever, M.A.; Išgum, I. Generative adversarial networks for noise reduction in low-dose CT. *IEEE Trans. Med. Imaging* **2017**, *36*, 2536–2545. [CrossRef] [PubMed]
14. Kang, E.; Min, J.; Ye, J.C. A deep convolutional neural network using directional wavelets for low-dose X-ray CT reconstruction. *Med. Phys.* **2017**, *44*, e360–e375. [CrossRef]
15. Mookiah, M.R.K.; Subburaj, K.; Mei, K.; Kopp, F.K.; Kaesmacher, J.; Jungmann, P.M.; Foehr, P.; Noel, P.B.; Kirschke, J.S.; Baum, T. Multidetector Computed Tomography Imaging: Effect of Sparse Sampling and Iterative Reconstruction on Trabecular Bone Microstructure. *J. Comput. Assist. Tomogr.* **2018**, *42*, 441–447. [CrossRef] [PubMed]
16. Nakamura, Y.; Higaki, T.; Tatsugami, F.; Zhou, J.; Yu, Z.; Akino, N.; Ito, Y.; Iida, M.; Awai, K. Deep Learning–based CT Image Reconstruction: Initial Evaluation Targeting Hypovascular Hepatic Metastases. *Radiol. Artif. Intell.* **2019**, *1*, e180011. [CrossRef]
17. Blau, Y.; Michaeli, T.; Israel, T. The Perception-Distortion Tradeoff Yochai. *Proc. IEEE Conf. Comput. Vis. Pattern Recognit.* **2018**, 6228–6237. [CrossRef]

18. Clark, K.; Vendt, B.; Smith, K.; Freymann, J.; Kirby, J.; Koppel, P.; Moore, S.; Phillips, S.; Maffitt, D.; Pringle, M.; et al. The cancer imaging archive (TCIA): Maintaining and operating a public information repository. *J. Digit. Imaging* **2013**, *26*, 1045–1057. [CrossRef]
19. TCGA-OV. Available online: http://doi.org/10.7937/K9/TCIA.2016.NDO1MDFQ (accessed on 20 December 2019).
20. TCGA Attribution. Available online: http://cancergenome.nih.gov/ (accessed on 20 December 2019).
21. Van Aarle, W.; Palenstijn, W.J.; Cant, J.; Janssens, E.; Bleichrodt, F.; Dabravolski, A.; De Beenhouwer, J.; Joost Batenburg, K.; Sijbers, J. Fast and flexible X-ray tomography using the ASTRA toolbox. *Opt. Express* **2016**, *24*, 25129. [CrossRef]
22. Van Aarle, W.; Palenstijn, W.J.; De Beenhouwer, J.; Altantzis, T.; Bals, S.; Batenburg, K.J.; Sijbers, J. The ASTRA Toolbox: A platform for advanced algorithm development in electron tomography. *Ultramicroscopy* **2015**, *157*, 35–47. [CrossRef]
23. Wang, Z.; Bovik, C.; Sheikh, H.R.; Simoncelli, E.P. Image Quality Assessment: From Error Visibility to Structural Similarity. *IEEE Trans. Image Process.* **2004**, *13*, 600–612. [CrossRef] [PubMed]
24. Fedorov, A.; Beichel, R.; Kalpathy-Cramer, J.; Finet, J.; Fillion-Robin, J.-C.; Pujol, S.; Jennings, D.; Bauer, C.; Sonka, M.; Fennessy, F. 3D Slicer as an Image Computing Platform for the Quantitative Imaging Network. *Magn. Reson. Imaging* **2012**, *30*, 1323–1341. [CrossRef]
25. Nougaret, S.; Addley, H.C.; Colombo, P.E.; Fujii, S.; Al Sharif, S.S.; Tirumani, S.H.; Jardon, K.; Sala, E.; Reinhold, C. Ovarian carcinomatosis: How the radiologist can help plan the surgical approach. *Radiographics* **2012**, *32*, 1775–1800. [CrossRef] [PubMed]
26. Eisenhauer, E.A.; Therasse, P.; Bogaerts, J.; Schwartz, L.H.; Sargent, D.; Ford, R.; Dancey, J.; Arbuck, S.; Gwyther, S.; Mooney, M.; et al. New response evaluation criteria in solid tumours: Revised RECIST guideline (version 1.1). *Eur. J. Cancer* **2009**, *45*, 228–247. [CrossRef] [PubMed]
27. Mutch, D.G.; Prat, J. 2014 FIGO staging for ovarian, fallopian tube and peritoneal cancer. *Gynecol. Oncol.* **2014**, *133*, 401–404. [CrossRef]
28. Akagi, M.; Nakamura, Y.; Higaki, T.; Narita, K.; Honda, Y.; Zhou, J.; Yu, Z.; Akino, N.; Awai, K. Deep learning reconstruction improves image quality of abdominal ultra-high-resolution CT. *Eur. Radiol.* **2019**, *29*, 6163–6171. [CrossRef]
29. Jin, S.O.; Kim, J.G.; Lee, S.Y.; Kwon, O.K. Bone-induced streak artifact suppression in sparse-view CT image reconstruction. *Biomed. Eng. Online* **2012**, *11*, 1–13. [CrossRef]
30. Du Bois, A.; Reuss, A.; Pujade-Lauraine, E.; Harter, P.; Ray-Coquard, I.; Pfisterer, J. Role of surgical outcome as prognostic factor in advanced epithelial ovarian cancer: A combined exploratory analysis of 3 prospectively randomized phase 3 multicenter trials: By the arbeitsgemeinschaft gynaekologische onkologie studiengruppe ovarialkarzin. *Cancer* **2009**, *115*, 1234–1244. [CrossRef]
31. Faure Conter, C.; Xia, C.; Gershenson, D.; Hurteau, J.; Covens, A.; Pashankar, F.; Krailo, M.; Billmire, D.; Patte, C.; Fresneau, B.; et al. Ovarian yolk sac tumors; does age matter? *Int. J. Gynecol. Cancer* **2018**, *28*, 77–84. [CrossRef]

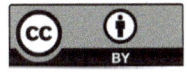

© 2020 by the authors. Licensee MDPI, Basel, Switzerland. This article is an open access article distributed under the terms and conditions of the Creative Commons Attribution (CC BY) license (http://creativecommons.org/licenses/by/4.0/).

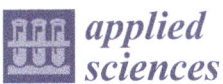

Article

Automatic Pancreas Segmentation Using Coarse-Scaled 2D Model of Deep Learning: Usefulness of Data Augmentation and Deep U-Net

Mizuho Nishio [1,*], Shunjiro Noguchi [1] and Koji Fujimoto [2]

1. Department of Diagnostic Imaging and Nuclear Medicine, Kyoto University Graduate School of Medicine, 54 Kawahara-cho, Shogoin, Sakyo-ku, Kyoto 606-8507, Japan; shunjiro101@gmail.com
2. Human Brain Research Center, Kyoto University Graduate School of Medicine, 54 Kawahara-cho, Shogoin, Sakyo-ku, Kyoto 606-8507, Japan; kfb@kuhp.kyoto-u.ac.jp
* Correspondence: nmizuho@kuhp.kyoto-u.ac.jp; Tel.: +81-75-751-3760; Fax: +81-75-771-9709

Received: 27 March 2020; Accepted: 9 May 2020; Published: 12 May 2020

Abstract: Combinations of data augmentation methods and deep learning architectures for automatic pancreas segmentation on CT images are proposed and evaluated. Images from a public CT dataset of pancreas segmentation were used to evaluate the models. Baseline U-net and deep U-net were chosen for the deep learning models of pancreas segmentation. Methods of data augmentation included conventional methods, mixup, and random image cropping and patching (RICAP). Ten combinations of the deep learning models and the data augmentation methods were evaluated. Four-fold cross validation was performed to train and evaluate these models with data augmentation methods. The dice similarity coefficient (DSC) was calculated between automatic segmentation results and manually annotated labels and these were visually assessed by two radiologists. The performance of the deep U-net was better than that of the baseline U-net with mean DSC of 0.703–0.789 and 0.686–0.748, respectively. In both baseline U-net and deep U-net, the methods with data augmentation performed better than methods with no data augmentation, and mixup and RICAP were more useful than the conventional method. The best mean DSC was obtained using a combination of deep U-net, mixup, and RICAP, and the two radiologists scored the results from this model as good or perfect in 76 and 74 of the 82 cases.

Keywords: pancreas; segmentation; computed tomography; deep learning; data augmentation

1. Introduction

Identification of anatomical structures is a fundamental step for radiologists in the interpretation of medical images. Similarly, automatic and accurate organ identification or segmentation is important for medical image analysis, computer-aided detection, and computer-aided diagnosis. To date, many studies have worked on automatic and accurate segmentation of organs, including lung, liver, pancreas, uterus, and muscle [1–5].

An estimated 606,880 Americans were predicted to die from cancer in 2019, in which 45,750 deaths would be due to pancreatic cancer [6]. Among all major types of cancers, the five-year relative survival rate of pancreatic cancer was the lowest (9%). One of the reasons for this low survival rate is the difficulty in the detection of pancreatic cancer in its early stages, because the organ is located in the retroperitoneal space and is in close proximity to other organs. A lack of symptoms is another reason for the difficulty of its early detection. Therefore, computer-aided detection and/or diagnosis using computed tomography (CT) may contribute to a reduction in the number of deaths caused by pancreatic cancer, similar to the effect of CT screenings on lung cancer [7,8]. Accurate segmentation of pancreas is the first step in the computer-aided detection/diagnosis system of pancreatic cancer.

Compared with conventional techniques of organ segmentation, which use hand-tuned filters and classifiers, deep learning, such as convolutional neural networks (CNN), is a framework, which lets computers learn and build these filters and classifiers from a huge amount of data. Recently, deep learning has been attracting much attention in medical image analysis, as it has been demonstrated as a powerful tool for organ segmentation [9]. Pancreas segmentation using CT images is challenging because the pancreas does not have a distinct border with its surrounding structures. In addition, pancreas has a large shape and size variability among people. Therefore, several different approaches to pancreas segmentation using deep learning have been proposed [10–15].

Previous studies designed to improve the deep learning model of automatic pancreas segmentation [10–15] can be classified using three major aspects: (i) dimension of the convolutional network, two-dimensional model (2D) versus three-dimensional model (3D); (ii) use of coarse-scaled model versus fine-scaled model; (iii) improvement of network architecture. In (i), the accuracy of pancreas segmentation was improved in a 3D model and compared with a 2D model; the 3D model makes it possible to fully utilize the 3D spatial information of pancreas, which is useful for grasping the large variability in pancreas shape and size. In (ii), an initial coarse-scaled model was used to obtain a rough region of interest (ROI) of the pancreas, and then the ROI was used for segmentation refinement using a fine-scaled model of pancreas segmentation. The difference in mean dice similarity coefficient (DSC) between the coarse-scaled and find-scaled models ranged from 2% to 7%. In (iii), the network architecture of a deep learning model was modified for efficient segmentation. For example, when an attention unit was introduced in a U-net, the segmentation accuracy was better than in a conventional U-net [12].

In previous studies, the usefulness of data augmentation in pancreas segmentation was not fully evaluated; only conventional methods of data augmentation were utilized. Recently proposed methods of data augmentation, such as mixup [16] and random image cropping and patching (RICAP) [17], were not evaluated.

In conventional data augmentation, horizontal flipping, vertical flipping, scaling, rotation, etc., are commonly used. It is necessary to find an effective combination of these, since among the possible combinations, some degrade the performance. Due to the number of the combinations, it is relatively cumbersome to eliminate the counterproductive combinations in conventional data augmentation. For this purpose, AutoAugment finds the best combination of data augmentation [18]. However, it is computationally expensive due to its use of reinforcement learning. In this regard, mixup and RICAP are easier to adjust than conventional data augmentation because they both have only one parameter.

The purpose of the current study is to evaluate and validate the combinations of different types of data augmentation and network architecture modification of U-net [19]. A deep U-net was used, to evaluate the usefulness of network architecture modification of U-net.

2. Materials and Methods

The current study used anonymized data extracted from a public database. Therefore, institutional review board approval was waived.

2.1. Dataset

The public dataset (Pancreas-CT) used in the current study includes 82 sets of contrast-enhanced abdominal CT images, where pancreas was manually annotated slice-by-slice [20,21]. This dataset is publicly available from The Cancer Imaging Archive [22]. The Pancreas-CT dataset is commonly used to benchmark the segmentation accuracy of pancreas on CT images. The CT scans in the dataset were obtained from 53 male and 27 female subjects. The age of the subjects ranged from 18 to 76 years with a mean age of 46.8 ± 16.7. The CT images were acquired with Philips and Siemens multi-detector CT scanners (120 kVp tube voltage). Spatial resolution of the CT images is 512 × 512 pixels with varying pixel sizes, and slice thickness is between 1.5–2.5 mm. As a part of image preprocessing, the pixel values for all sets of CT images were clipped to [−100, 240] Hounsfield units, then rescaled to the range [0, 1]. This preprocessing was commonly used for the Pancreas-CT dataset [15].

2.2. Deep Learning Model

U-net was used as a baseline model of deep learning in the current study [19]. U-net consists of encoding–decoding architecture. Downsampling and upsampling are performed in the encoding and decoding parts of U-net, respectively. The most important characteristic of U-net is the presence of shortcut connections between the encoding part and the decoding part at equal resolution. While the baseline U-net performs downsampling and upsampling 4 times [19], deep U-net performs downsampling and upsampling 6 times. In addition to the number of downsampling and upsampling, the number of feature maps in the convolution layer and the use of dropout were changed in the deep U-net; the number of feature maps in the first convolution layer equaled to 40 and dropout probability to 2%. In the baseline U-net, 64 feature maps and no dropout were used. In both, the baseline U-net and the deep U-net, the number of feature maps in the convolution layer was doubled after each downsampling. Figure 1 presents the deep U-net model of the proposed method. Both the baseline U-net and deep U-net utilized batch normalization. Keras (https://keras.io/) with Tensorflow (https://www.tensorflow.org/) backends was used for the implementation of the U-net models. Image dimension of the input and output in the two U-net models was 512 × 512 pixels.

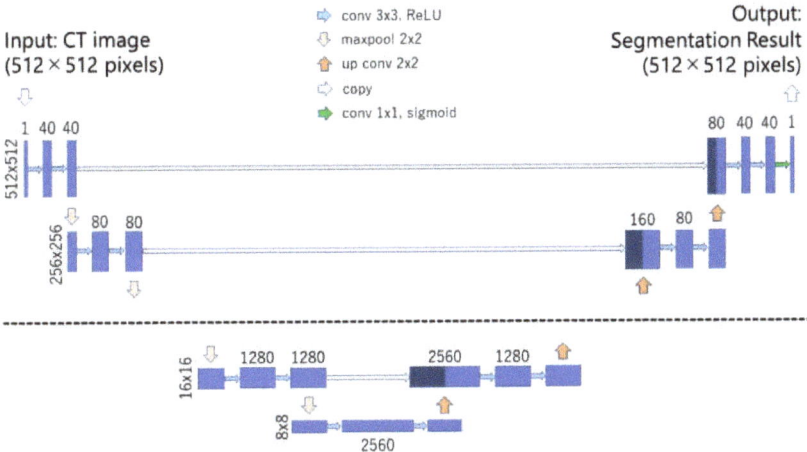

Figure 1. Illustration of the deep U-net model. The number of downsampling and upsampling is 6 in the deep U-net. Except for the last convolution layer, dropout and convolution layer are coupled. Abbreviations: convolution layer (conv), maxpooling layer (maxpool), upsampling and convolution layer (up conv), rectified linear unit (ReLU).

2.3. Data Augmentation

To prevent overfitting in the training of the deep learning model, we utilized the following three types of data augmentation methods: conventional method, mixup [16], and RICAP [17]. Although mixup and RICAP were initially proposed for image classification tasks, we utilized them for segmentation by merging or cropping/patching labels in the same way as is done for images.

Conventional augmentation methods included ±5° rotation, ±5% x-axis shift, ±5% y-axis shift, and 95%–105% scaling. Both image and label were changed by the same transformation when using a conventional augmentation method.

Mixup generates a new training sample from linear combination of existing images and their labels [16]. Here, two sets of training samples are denoted by (x, y) and (x', y'), where x and x' are images, and y and y' are their labels. A generated sample $(x^\#, y^\#)$ is given by:

$$x^\# = \lambda x + (1 - \lambda) x' \qquad (1)$$

$$y^\# = \lambda y + (1 - \lambda) y' \qquad (2)$$

where λ ranges from 0 to 1 and is distributed according to beta distribution: $\lambda \sim Beta(\beta, \beta)$ for $\beta \in (0, \infty)$. The two samples to be combined are selected randomly from the training data. The hyperparameter β of mixup was set to 0.2 empirically.

RICAP generates a new training sample from four randomly selected images [17]. The four images are randomly cropped and patched according to a boundary position (w, h), which is determined according to beta distribution: $w \sim Beta(\beta, \beta)$ and $h \sim Beta(\beta, \beta)$. We set the hyperparameter β of RICAP to 0.4 empirically. For four images to be combined, the coordinates (x_k, y_k) ($k = 1, 2, 3,$ and 4) of the upper left corners of the cropped areas are randomly selected. The sizes of the four cropped images are determined based on the value (w, h), such that they do not increase the original image size. A generated sample is obtained by combining the four cropped images. In the current study, the image and its label were cropped at the same coordinate and size.

2.4. Training

Dice loss function was used as the optimization target of the deep learning models. RMSprop was used as the optimizer, and its learning rate was set to 0.00004. The number of training epochs was set to 45. Following previous works on pancreas segmentation, we used 4-fold cross-validation to assess the robustness of the model (20 or 21 subjects were chosen for validation in folds). The hyperparameters related with U-net and its training were selected using random search [23]. After the random search, the hyperparameters were fixed. The following 10 combinations of deep learning models and data augmentation methods were used:

1. Baseline U-net + no data augmentation,
2. Baseline U-net + conventional method,
3. Baseline U-net + mixup,
4. Baseline U-net + RICAP,
5. Baseline U-net + RICAP + mixup,
6. Deep U-net + no data augmentation,
7. Deep U-net + conventional method,
8. Deep U-net + mixup,
9. Deep U-net + RICAP,
10. Deep U-net + RICAP + mixup.

2.5. Evaluation of Pancreas Segmentation

For each validation case of the Pancreas-CT dataset, three-dimensional CT images were processed slice-by-slice using the trained deep learning models, and the segmentation results were stacked. Except for the stacking, no complex postprocessing was utilized. Quantitative and qualitative evaluations were performed for the automatic segmentation results.

The metrics of quantitative evaluation were calculated using the three-dimensional segmentation results and annotated labels. Four types of metrics were used for the quantitative evaluation of the segmentation results: dice similarity coefficient (DSC), Jaccard index (JI), sensitivity (SE), and specificity (SP). These metrics are defined by the following equations:

$$DSC = \frac{2|P \cap L|}{|P| + |L|} \quad (3)$$

$$JI = \frac{|P \cap L|}{|P| + |L| - |P \cap L|} \quad (4)$$

$$SE = \frac{|P \cap L|}{|L|} \quad (5)$$

$$SP = 1 - \frac{|P| - |P \cap L|}{|I| - |L|} \quad (6)$$

where $|P|$, $|L|$, and $|I|$ denote the number of voxels for pancreas segmentation results, annotated label of pancreas segmentation, and three-dimensional CT images, respectively. $|P \cap L|$ represents the number of voxels where the deep learning models can accurately segment pancreas (true positive). Before calculating the four metrics, a threshold of 0.5 was used for obtaining pancreas segmentation mask from the output of the U-net [24]. The threshold of 0.5 was fixed for all the 82 cases. A Wilcoxon signed rank test was used to test statistical significance among the DSC results of 10 combinations of deep learning models and data augmentation methods. Bonferroni correction was used for controlling family wise error rate. p-values less than $0.05/45 = 0.00111$ was considered as statistical significance.

For the qualitative evaluation, two radiologists with 14 and 6 years of experience visually evaluated both the manually annotated labels and automatic segmentation results using a 5-point scale: 1, unacceptable; 2, slightly unacceptable; 3, acceptable; 4, good; 5, perfect. Inter-observer variability between the two radiologists were evaluated using weighted kappa with squared weight.

3. Results

Table 1 shows results of the qualitative evaluation of the pancreas segmentation of Deep U-net + RICAP + mixup and the manually annotated labels. The mean visual scores of manually annotated labels were 4.951 and 4.902 for the two radiologists, and those of automatic segmentation results were 4.439 and 4.268. The mean score of automatic segmentation results demonstrates that the accuracy of the automatic segmentation was good; more than 92.6% (76/82) and 87.8% (74/82) of the cases were scored as 4 or above. Notably, Table 1 shows that the manually annotated labels were scored as 4 (good, but not perfect) in four and eight cases by the two radiologists. Weighted kappa values between the two radiologists were 0.465 (moderate agreement) for the manually annotated labels and 0.723 (substantial agreement) for the automatic segmentation results.

Table 1. Results of qualitative evaluation of automatic pancreas segmentation and manually annotated labels.

Radiologist	Target	Number of Score 1	Number of Score 2	Number of Score 3	Number of Score 4	Number of Score 5
Radiologist 1	manually annotated label	0	0	0	4	78
Radiologist 1	automatic segmentation	0	3	3	31	45
Radiologist 2	manually annotated label	0	0	0	8	74
Radiologist 2	automatic segmentation	0	2	6	42	32

Table 2 shows the results of the quantitative evaluation of pancreas segmentation. Mean and standard deviation of DSC, JI, SE, and SP are calculated from the validation cases of 4-fold cross validation for the Pancreas-CT dataset. Mean DSC of the deep U-net (0.703–0.789) was better than the mean DSC of the baseline U-net (0.686–0.748) across all data augmentation methods. Because mean SP was 1.00 in all the combinations, non-pancreas lesions were not segmented by the models. Therefore, mean DSC was mainly affected by mean SE (segmentation accuracy only for pancreas lesion) as shown in Table 2. Table 2 also shows the usefulness of data augmentation. In both, the baseline U-net and deep U-net, the model combined with any of the three types of data augmentation performed better than the model with no data augmentation. In addition, mixup and RICAP were more useful than the conventional method; the best mean DSC was obtained using the combination of mixup and RICAP. The best mean DSC was obtained using the deep U-net with RICAP and mixup.

Table 2. Results of quantitative evaluation of automatic pancreas segmentation from the 82 cases using 4-fold cross validation.

Type of Model and Data Augmentation	DSC	JI	SE	SP
Baseline U-net + no data augmentation	0.686 ± 0.186	0.548 ± 0.186	0.618 ± 0.221	1.000 ± 0.000
Baseline U-net + conventional method	0.694 ± 0.182	0.556 ± 0.183	0.631 ± 0.220	1.000 ± 0.000
Baseline U-net + mixup	0.733 ± 0.106	0.588 ± 0.122	0.698 ± 0.155	1.000 ± 0.000
Baseline U-net + RICAP	0.699 ± 0.155	0.557 ± 0.169	0.624 ± 0.200	1.000 ± 0.000
Baseline U-net + RICAP + mixup	0.748 ± 0.127	0.611 ± 0.141	0.700 ± 0.176	1.000 ± 0.000
Deep U-net + no data augmentation	0.703 ± 0.166	0.563 ± 0.169	0.645 ± 0.201	1.000 ± 0.000
Deep U-net + conventional method	0.720 ± 0.171	0.586 ± 0.176	0.685 ± 0.210	1.000 ± 0.000
Deep U-net + mixup	0.725 ± 0.125	0.582 ± 0.137	0.694 ± 0.158	1.000 ± 0.000
Deep U-net + RICAP	0.740 ± 0.160	0.609 ± 0.169	0.691 ± 0.200	1.000 ± 0.000
Deep U-net + RICAP + mixup	0.789 ± 0.083	0.658 ± 0.103	0.762 ± 0.120	1.000 ± 0.000

Note: data are shown as mean ± standard deviation. Abbreviations: Random image cropping and patching (RICAP), dice similarity coefficient (DSC), Jaccard index (JI), sensitivity (SE), and specificity (SP).

Table A2 of Appendix B shows the results of the Wilcoxon signed rank test. After the Bonferroni correction, the DSC differences between Deep U-net + RICAP + mixup and the other six models were statistically significant.

Representative images of pancreas segmentation are shown in Figures 2 and 3. In the case of Figure 2, the manually annotated label was scored as 4 by the two radiologists because the main pancreas duct and its surrounding tissue were excluded from the label.

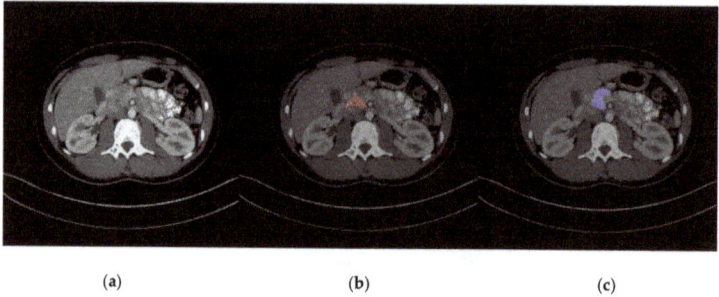

(a) (b) (c)

Figure 2. Representative image of automatic pancreas segmentation. (a) Original computed tomography (CT) image; (b) CT image with manually annotated label in red, scored as not perfect by two radiologists; (c) CT image with automatic segmentation in blue.

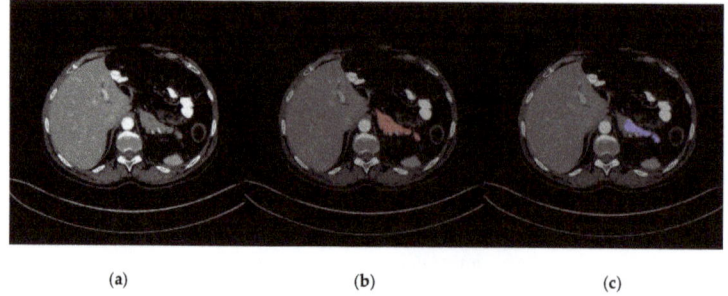

(a) (b) (c)

Figure 3. Representative image of a low-quality automatic pancreas segmentation. (a) Original computed tomography (CT) image; (b) CT image with manually annotated label in red; (c) CT image with automatic segmentation in blue, with part of the pancreas excluded from the segmentation.

4. Discussion

The results of the present study show that the three types of data augmentation were useful for the pancreas segmentation in both the baseline U-net and deep U-net. In addition, the deep U-net, which is characterized by additional layers, was overall more effective for automatic pancreas segmentation than the baseline U-net. In data augmentation, not only the conventional method, but also mixup and RICAP were useful for pancreas segmentation; the combination of mixup and RICAP was the most useful.

Table 3 summarizes results of previous studies using the Pancreas-CT dataset. While Table 3 includes the studies with coarse-scaled models, Table A1 includes the studies with fine-scaled models. As shown in Table 3, the coarse-scaled 2D model of the current study achieved sufficiently high accuracy, comparable to those of previous studies. While the present study focused on the 2D coarse-scaled models, the data augmentation methods used in the present study can be easily applied to 3D fine-scaled models. Therefore, it can be expected that the combination of the proposed data augmentation methods and 3D fine-scaled models might lead to further improvement of automatic pancreas segmentation.

Table 3. Summary of coarse-scaled models using the Pancreas-CT dataset.

Name of Model	2D/3D	Coarse/Fine	Mean DSC	Data Splitting
Holistically Nested 2D FCN Stage-1 [11]	2D	coarse	0.768 ± 0.111	4-fold CV
2D FCN [13]	2D	coarse	0.803 ± 0.09	4-fold CV
Coarse-scaled Model 2D FCN [14]	2D	coarse	0.757 ± 0.105	4-fold CV
Single Model 3D U-net [12] (trained from scratch)	3D	coarse	0.815 ± 0.057	61 training and 21 test sets randomly selected
Single Model 3D Attention U-net [12] (trained from scratch)	3D	coarse	0.821 ± 0.068	61 training and 21 test sets randomly selected
Coarse-scaled Model 3D U-net [15]	3D	coarse	0.819 ± 0.068	4-fold CV
Proposed model	2D	coarse	0.789 ± 0.083	4-fold CV

Data augmentation was originally proposed for the classification model, and the effectiveness of mixup was validated for segmentation on brain MRI images [25]. The results of the current study demonstrate the effectiveness of multiple types of data augmentation methods for the two models of U-net for automatic pancreatic segmentation. To the best of our knowledge, the current study is the first to validate the usefulness of multiple types of data augmentation methods in pancreas segmentation.

Table 2 shows that deep U-net was better than baseline U-net. Deep U-net included additional layers in its network architecture, compared with baseline U-net. It is speculated that these additional layers could lead to performance improvement for pancreas segmentation. Nakai et al. [26] showed that deeper U-net could efficiently denoised low-dose CT images. They also showed that deeper U-net was better than baseline U-net. Kurata et al. [4] showed that their U-net with additional layers was effective for uterine segmentation. The results of the current study are consistent with the results of these studies. The effectiveness of deep/deeper U-net has not been sufficiently investigated so far. Because U-net can be used for segmentation, image denoising, detection, and modality conversion, it is necessary to evaluate what tasks the deep/deeper U-net is effective for.

Combined use of mixup and RICAP was the best for data augmentation in the current study. The combination of mixup and RICAP was also used in the study of bone segmentation [24]. The results of bone segmentation show that effectiveness of data augmentation was observed in the dataset with limited cases, and the optimal combination was conventional method and RICAP. Based on the studies of bone and pancreas segmentation, usefulness of combination of conventional method, mixup, and RICAP should be further investigated.

Sandfort et al. used CycleGAN as data augmentation to improve generalizability in organ segmentation on CT images [27]. CycleGAN was also used for data augmentation in the classification task [28]. Because the computational cost of training CycleGAN is relatively high, the use of CycleGAN as a data augmentation method needs some consideration. In this regard, computational cost of mixup and RICAP is relatively low, and mixup and RICAP are easy to implement.

Accuracy of pancreas segmentation was visually evaluated by the two radiologists in the current study. To our knowledge, there was no study of deep learning to evaluate the segmentation accuracy of pancreas structure visually. The results of visual scores mean that automatic segmentation model of the current study was good. It is expected that the proposed model may be useful for clinical cases if the clinical CT images have similar condition and quality to those of the Pancreas-CT dataset.

In the current study, we evaluated automatic pancreas segmentation using the public dataset called Pancreas-CT. Although this dataset was used in several studies as shown in Table 3, the manually annotated labels of four or eight cases were scored as not perfect based on the visual assessment of the current study. In most of the cases, the labels for the pancreas head were assessed as low-quality. It is presumed that the low-quality labeling is caused by the fact that annotators did not fully understand the boundary between the pancreas and other organs (e.g., duodenum). To evaluate the segmentation accuracy, reliable labeling is mandatory. For this purpose, a new database for pancreas segmentation is desirable.

There were several limitations to the present study. First, we investigated the usefulness of data augmentation only in segmentation models. The usefulness of data augmentation should be evaluated for other models such as classification, detection, and image generation. Second, the 3D fine-tuned model of pancreas segmentation was not evaluated. Because U-net, mixup, and RICAP were originally suggested for 2D models, we constructed and evaluated the 2D model of pancreas segmentation. We will apply the proposed methods to the 3D fine-tuned model in future research.

5. Conclusions

The combination of deep U-net with mixup and RICAP achieved automatic pancreas segmentation, which the radiologists scored as good or perfect. We will further investigate the usefulness of the proposed method for the 3D coarse-scaled/fine-scaled models to improve segmentation accuracy.

Author Contributions: Conceptualization, M.N.; methodology, M.N.; software, M.N. and S.N.; validation, M.N. and S.N.; formal analysis, M.N.; investigation, M.N.; resources, M.N. and K.F.; data curation, M.N. and SN; writing—original draft preparation, M.N.; writing—review and editing, M.N., S.N., and K.F.; visualization, M.N.; supervision, K.F.; project administration, M.N.; funding acquisition, M.N. All authors have read and agreed to the published version of the manuscript.

Funding: The present study was supported by JSPS KAKENHI, grant number JP19K17232.

Conflicts of Interest: The authors declare no conflict of interest. The funders had no role in the design of the study; in the collection, analyses, or interpretation of data; in the writing of the manuscript, or in the decision to publish the results.

Appendix A

Table A1. Summary of fine-scaled models using Pancreas-CT dataset.

Name of Model	2D/3D	Coarse/Fine	Mean DSC	Data Splitting
Holistically Nested 2D FCN Stage-2 [11]	2D	fine	0.811 ± 0.073	4-fold CV
2D FCN + Recurrent Network [13]	2D	fine	0.824 ± 0.067	4-fold CV
Fine-scaled Model 2D FCN [14]	2D	fine	0.824 ± 0.057	4-fold CV
Fine-scaled Model 3D U-net [15]	3D	fine	0.860 ± 0.045	4-fold CV

Appendix B

Table A2. Results of Statistical significance for DSC difference.

Target 1	Target 2	p-Value	Statistical Significance for DSC Difference
1	2	0.727381623	No
1	3	0.560489877	No
1	4	0.921405534	No
1	5	0.037061458	No
1	6	0.727381623	No
1	7	0.148802462	No
1	8	0.553863735	No
1	9	0.012907274	No
1	10	5.45×10^{-5}	Yes
2	3	0.85904175	No
2	4	0.87456599	No
2	5	0.080182031	No
2	6	0.958034301	No
2	7	0.211395881	No
2	8	0.856459499	No
2	9	0.029961825	No
2	10	0.000143632	Yes
3	4	0.422285602	No
3	5	0.057745373	No
3	6	0.668985055	No
3	7	0.331951771	No
3	8	0.85904175	No
3	9	0.033624033	No
3	10	3.72×10^{-5}	Yes
4	5	0.047352438	No
4	6	0.764727204	No
4	7	0.157310432	No
4	8	0.529901132	No
4	9	0.024270868	No
4	10	0.000120757	Yes
5	6	0.067465313	No
5	7	0.649935631	No
5	8	0.067465313	No
5	9	0.580595554	No
5	10	0.031228349	No
6	7	0.227439002	No
6	8	0.784877257	No
6	9	0.028739708	No
6	10	9.60×10^{-5}	Yes
7	8	0.292611693	No
7	9	0.355409719	No
7	10	0.017108607	No
8	9	0.040470933	No
8	10	5.23×10^{-5}	Yes
9	10	0.185045722	No

Note: In Target 1 and Target 2, values of cells mean the followings: (1) Baseline U-net + no data augmentation, (2) Baseline U-net + conventional method, (3) Baseline U-net + mixup, (4) Baseline U-net + RICAP, (5) Baseline U-net + RICAP + mixup, (6) Deep U-net + no data augmentation, (7) Deep U-net + conventional method, (8) Deep U-net + mixup, (9) Deep U-net + RICAP, (10) Deep U-net + RICAP + mixup. p-values less than 0.05/45 = 0.00111 was considered as statistical significance.

References

1. Nakagomi, K.; Shimizu, A.; Kobatake, H.; Yakami, M.; Fujimoto, K.; Togashi, K. Multi-shape graph cuts with neighbor prior constraints and its application to lung segmentation from a chest CT volume. *Med. Image Anal.* **2013**, *17*, 62–77. [CrossRef] [PubMed]
2. Seo, H.; Huang, C.; Bassenne, M.; Xiao, R.; Xing, L. Modified U-Net (mU-Net) with Incorporation of Object-Dependent High Level Features for Improved Liver and Liver-Tumor Segmentation in CT Images. *IEEE Trans. Med. Imaging* **2020**, *39*, 1316–1325. [CrossRef] [PubMed]
3. Asaturyan, H.; Gligorievski, A.; Villarini, B. Morphological and multi-level geometrical descriptor analysis in CT and MRI volumes for automatic pancreas segmentation. *Comput. Med. Imaging Graph.* **2019**, *75*, 1–13. [CrossRef] [PubMed]
4. Kurata, Y.; Nishio, M.; Kido, A.; Fujimoto, K.; Yakami, M.; Isoda, H.; Togashi, K. Automatic segmentation of the uterus on MRI using a convolutional neural network. *Comput. Biol. Med.* **2019**, *114*, 103438. [CrossRef] [PubMed]
5. Hiasa, Y.; Otake, Y.; Takao, M.; Ogawa, T.; Sugano, N.; Sato, Y. Automated Muscle Segmentation from Clinical CT using Bayesian U-Net for Personalized Musculoskeletal Modeling. *IEEE Trans. Med. Imaging* **2020**, *39*, 1030–1040. [CrossRef]
6. Siegel, R.L.; Miller, K.D.; Jemal, A. Cancer statistics, 2019. *CA Cancer J. Clin.* **2019**, *69*, 7–34. [CrossRef] [PubMed]
7. Ardila, D.; Kiraly, A.P.; Bharadwaj, S.; Choi, B.; Reicher, J.J.; Peng, L.; Tse, D.; Etemadi, M.; Ye, W.; Corrado, G.; et al. End-to-end lung cancer screening with three-dimensional deep learning on low-dose chest computed tomography. *Nat. Med.* **2019**, *25*, 954–961. [CrossRef] [PubMed]
8. National Lung Screening Trial Research Team; Aberle, D.R.; Adams, A.M.; Berg, C.D.; Black, W.C.; Clapp, J.D.; Fagerstrom, R.M.; Gareen, I.F.; Gatsonis, C.; Marcus, P.M.; et al. Reduced lung-cancer mortality with low-dose computed tomographic screening. *N. Engl. J. Med.* **2011**, *365*, 395–409.
9. Hesamian, M.H.; Jia, W.; He, X.; Kennedy, P. Deep Learning Techniques for Medical Image Segmentation: Achievements and Challenges. *J. Digit. Imaging* **2019**, *32*, 582–596. [CrossRef]
10. Kumar, H.; DeSouza, S.V.; Petrov, M.S. Automated pancreas segmentation from computed tomography and magnetic resonance images: A systematic review. *Comput. Methods Programs Biomed.* **2019**, *178*, 319–328. [CrossRef]
11. Roth, H.R.; Lu, L.; Lay, N.; Harrison, A.P.; Farag, A.; Sohn, A.; Summers, R.M. Spatial aggregation of holistically-nested convolutional neural networks for automated pancreas localization and segmentation. *Med. Image Anal.* **2018**, *45*, 94–107. [CrossRef] [PubMed]
12. Oktay, O.; Schlemper, J.; Folgoc, L.L.; Lee, M.; Heinrich, M.; Misawa, K.; Mori, K.; McDonagh, S.; Hammerla, N.Y.; Kainz, B.; et al. Attention U-Net: Learning Where to Look for the Pancreas. In Proceedings of the 1st Conference on Medical Imaging with Deep Learning (MIDL2018), Amsterdam, The Netherlands, 4–6 July 2018.
13. Cai, J.; Lu, L.; Xie, Y.; Xing, F.; Yang, L. Improving deep pancreas segmentation in CT and MRI images via recurrent neural contextual learning and direct loss function. In Proceedings of the MICCAI 2017, Quebec City, QC, Canada, 11–13 September 2017.
14. Zhou, Y.; Xie, L.; Shen, W.; Wang, Y.; Fishman, E.K.; Yuille, A.L. A fixed-point model for pancreas segmentation in abdominal CT scans. In Proceedings of the MICCAI 2017, Quebec City, QC, Canada, 11–13 September 2017.
15. Zhao, N.; Tong, N.; Ruan, D.; Sheng, K. Fully Automated Pancreas Segmentation with Two-stage 3D Convolutional Neural Networks. *arXiv* **2019**, arXiv:1906.01795.
16. Zhang, H.; Cisse, M.; Dauphin, Y.N.; Lopez-Paz, D. mixup: Beyond Empirical Risk Minimization. *arXiv* **2017**, arXiv:1710.09412.
17. Takahashi, R.; Matsubara, T.; Uehara, K. Data Augmentation using Random Image Cropping and Patching for Deep CNNs. *arXiv* **2018**, arXiv:1811.09030. [CrossRef]
18. Cubuk, E.D.; Zoph, B.; Mane, D.; Vasudevan, V.; Le, Q.V. AutoAugment: Learning Augmentation Policies from Data. In Proceedings of the Computer Vision and Pattern Recognition (CVPR2019), Long Beach, CA, USA, 16–20 June 2019.

19. Ronneberger, O.; Fischer, P.; Brox, T. U-net: Convolutional networks for biomedical image segmentation. In Proceedings of the International Conference on Medical Image Computing and Computer-Assisted Intervention, Munich, Germany, 5–9 October 2015; Volume 9351, pp. 234–241.
20. Roth, H.R.; Farag, A.; Turkbey, E.B.; Lu, L.; Liu, J.; Summers, R.M. Data from Pancreas-CT. The Cancer Imaging Archive. 2016. Available online: http://doi.org/10.7937/K9/TCIA.2016.tNB1kqBU (accessed on 13 February 2020).
21. Roth, H.R.; Lu, L.; Farag, A.; Shin, H.-C.; Liu, J.; Turkbey, E.B.; Summers, R.M. DeepOrgan: Multi-level Deep Convolutional Networks for Automated Pancreas Segmentation. In Proceedings of the MICCA 2015, Munich, Germany, 5–9 October 2015; Volume 9349, pp. 556–564.
22. Clark, K.; Vendt, B.; Smith, K.; Freymann, J.; Kirby, J.; Koppel, P.; Moore, S.; Phillips, S.; Maffitt, D.; Pringle, M.; et al. The Cancer Imaging Archive (TCIA): Maintaining and Operating a Public Information Repository. *J. Digit. Imaging* **2013**, *26*, 1045–1057. [CrossRef] [PubMed]
23. Bergstra, J.; Bardenet, R.; Bengio, Y.; Kégl, B. Algorithms for Hyper-Parameter Optimization. In Proceedings of the 25th Annual Conference on Neural Information Processing Systems 2011, Granada, Spain, 12–15 December 2011; Available online: http://dl.acm.org/citation.cfm?id=2986743 (accessed on 5 May 2020).
24. Noguchi, S.; Nishio, M.; Yakami, M.; Nakagomi, L.; Togashi, K. Bone segmentation on whole-body CT using convolutional neural network with novel data augmentation techniques. *Comput. Biol. Med.* **2020**, *121*, 103767. [CrossRef] [PubMed]
25. Eaton-Rosen, Z.; Bragman, F.; Ourselin, S.; Cardoso, M.J. Improving Data Augmentation for Medical Image Segmentation. In Proceedings of the 1st Conference on Medical Imaging with Deep Learning (MIDL 2018), Amsterdam, The Netherlands, 4–6 July 2018.
26. Nakai, H.; Nishio, M.; Yamashita, R.; Ono, A.; Nakao, K.K.; Fujimoto, K.; Togashi, K. Quantitative and Qualitative Evaluation of Convolutional Neural Networks with a Deeper U-Net for Sparse-View Computed Tomography Reconstruction. *Acad. Radiol.* **2020**, *27*, 563–574. [CrossRef] [PubMed]
27. Sandfort, V.; Yan, K.; Pickhardt, P.J.; Summers, R.M. Data augmentation using generative adversarial networks (CycleGAN) to improve generalizability in CT segmentation tasks. *Sci. Rep.* **2019**, *9*, 16884. [CrossRef] [PubMed]
28. Muramatsu, C.; Nishio, M.; Goto, T.; Oiwa, M.; Morita, T.; Yakami, M.; Kubo, T.; Togashi, K.; Fujita, H. Improving breast mass classification by shared data with domain transformation using a generative adversarial network. *Comput. Biol. Med.* **2020**, *119*, 103698. [CrossRef] [PubMed]

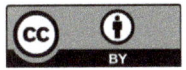

© 2020 by the authors. Licensee MDPI, Basel, Switzerland. This article is an open access article distributed under the terms and conditions of the Creative Commons Attribution (CC BY) license (http://creativecommons.org/licenses/by/4.0/).

MDPI
St. Alban-Anlage 66
4052 Basel
Switzerland
Tel. +41 61 683 77 34
Fax +41 61 302 89 18
www.mdpi.com

Applied Sciences Editorial Office
E-mail: applsci@mdpi.com
www.mdpi.com/journal/applsci

www.ingramcontent.com/pod-product-compliance
Lightning Source LLC
LaVergne TN
LVHW070555100526
838202LV00012B/479